LUST *for* LOVE

LUST *for* LOVE

Rekindling Intimacy *and* Passion *in your* Relationship

Pamela Anderson *and*
Rabbi Shmuley Boteach

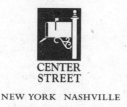

CENTER
STREET

NEW YORK NASHVILLE

Center Street
Hachette Book Group
1290 Avenue of the Americas, New York, NY 10104
centerstreet.com
twitter.com/centerstreet

First Edition: April 2018

Center Street is a division of Hachette Book Group, Inc. The Center Street name and logo are trademarks of Hachette Book Group, Inc.

The publisher is not responsible for websites (or their content) that are not owned by the publisher.

The Hachette Speakers Bureau provides a wide range of authors for speaking events. To find out more, go to www.HachetteSpeakersBureau.com or call (866) 376-6591.

Library of Congress Cataloging-in-Publication Data has been applied for.

LCCN: 2017959355

ISBNs: 978-1-4789-9278-3 (hardcover), 978-1-4789-9277-6 (ebook)

Printed in the United States of America

LSC-C

10 9 8 7 6 5 4 3 2 1

PAMELA ANDERSON:

For my wonderfully
spirited and talented boys.
Brandon and Dylan Lee
who were raised
by wolves,
with wisdom inspired by
ancient cultures,
mythology, music and art—
I admire your courage,
your independence
and the extreme faith you both have
in yourselves—
To be you
and no one else
is the hardest and most rewarding road.
I love you endlessly.

With pride,
Your wild and loving
Mom

RABBI SHMULEY BOTEACH:

To my sons-in-law Arik, Yossi, and Moshe
For loving my daughters and being real husband material

There are three things that are too amazing for me,
four that I do not understand:
the way of an eagle in the sky,
the way of a snake on a rock,
the way of a ship on the high seas,
and the way of a man with a young woman.

Proverbs 30:18–19

CONTENTS

Part Six:
PUTTING PASSION INTO PRACTICE

ACKNOWLEDGMENTS

PAMELA ANDERSON:

To the many friends, family and associates without whose help and support this work could not have come about: please accept my heartfelt gratitude and appreciation. Without you I could not have done this. Thank you.

RABBI SHMULEY BOTEACH:

Thank you to all the people who have discussed their relationships and marriages with me over three decades that has deepened my understanding of human nature and the essential ingredients of love, passion, intimacy, and romance. I thank you for your confidence and hope I made a positive difference in your lives. A giant thank you to my children who are my inspiration, happiness, and joy. The greatest debt of gratitude to my wife and soulmate Debbie who illuminates and brings blessing to all things. And the greatest debt of gratitude of all to God Almighty, Creator of heaven and earth, who created love and oneness, the glue that holds the universe together.

PREFACE BY

Pamela Anderson

When two people from radically different backgrounds agree wholeheartedly on something, listen closely. There is a good chance that what they have to say might just be important. Let this book be the proof of that. The co-authors of this book, Rabbi Shmuley Boteach and I, are indeed very different people, from very different traditions, and with very different approaches to life and the world. An outspoken, courageous, and prolific speaker and writer, Shmuley is also a religious teacher. The perspective he brings to *Lust for Love* is drawn from years of experience providing advice and counseling to married couples.

My background contrasts with Shmuley's. Many would consider it the opposite of his. But while the broad strokes of my biography are well known, there is also a private side of my life that few will have heard. I started modeling for *Playboy* at the age of twenty-two and spent my twenties as a cast member on *Baywatch*. At an age when most people are discovering themselves for the first time as adults—in a time before the Internet had yet taken over our lives and everyone had a taste of celebrity—I found myself sharing my own image with a generation. I watched as my name broke out from my immediate circle of friends, eventually reaching households all over the world. Surreally, I was called a "sex symbol," a "bombshell," a "goddess."

It was a disconcerting experience for a shy, small-town girl from Vancouver Island—a quiet, studious girl who loved her mom and dad but who also had to deal with no small amount of trauma. In the early days it was tough, grappling with uncertainty and the sense of exposure. But I discovered I felt comfortable as long as I pretended to be someone else—playing the part in public, finding within myself a different persona for every shoot.

Some might smirk, but in no way do I want to disown the *Playboy* years or diminish their importance to me. These experiences were a sort of university for me. Through them, I was given the opportunity to meet and befriend fascinating and beguiling people—men and women, souls and intellects—whose experiences and character and wisdom shaped me. It was an education—unique and brilliant and precious. Thinking of these years I am reminded of the words Anaïs Nin wrote on the development of woman on her own terms, rather than as an imitation of man. The theme of "woman finding her own language, articulating her own feelings, discovering her own perceptions."[1]

It's sometimes assumed that I should want to renounce those years as decadent or foolish. This is not the case. In hindsight, I am very proud of the independent, unorthodox path I took, a path that allowed me to develop on my own terms, and not—as some might presume—on the terms of men. I am proud of the intense spiritual rewards my life has brought me and the wisdom I have been lucky enough to receive.

Most of all, I am proud and in awe of the women I've met along the way—powerful, wise, fascinating women; women as diverse and varied, as contradictory and manifold, as the types Nin lists in her diaries: "the masculine, objective one; the child woman of the world; the maternal woman; the sensation-seeker; the unconsciously dramatic one; the churlish one; the cold, egotistical one; and the healing, intuitive guide-woman."[2]

I want to do justice to these women. I don't at all renounce my past. It is out of those experiences—and with these companions and guides— that I was able to define myself. It would have been so easy to lose myself then, eclipsed behind a stream of images. But I was there, among these women, and it is there I came to understand the power and autonomy that was available to me in sensuality, there that I came to possess myself in that power, and that is what saved me.

It hasn't all been roses. Over the years, I learned that fame can also be a prison. It can leave very little room for a real person to live behind it, very little space for honesty, and very little time to age, or mourn, or love. Life is untidier than celebrity makes out. At times in my life it has been hard to shake the sense that my life was happening to someone else—that I was the lesser twin to my public image: Pamela and me. It was Pamela who won the praise and the credit, renowned but shallow, never really allowed or expected to have any depth, while I was the thoughtful, sensitive one, reading voraciously, searching for meaning, suffering through my divorce and raising my boys, sometimes waking up and wondering where the last twenty years had gone.

"Look for something hard enough and you will find it," my father once told me. Lately, I have taken a hard look at my life and experiences, and I've realized that I have a lot to say. *Playboy* models aren't supposed to have much to say—at least according to some—but it is this very background that I draw on for my philosophy. That's why, when I first met Rabbi Shmuley Boteach, I did not expect that we would find so much to agree on.

I was introduced to Shmuley through mutual friends based in Malibu. He wanted to recognize my activism at the Champions of Jewish Values International Awards Gala. I was honored that I—having no Jewish background—would be recognized in this way. I went along, curious to meet him. Our first conversations were cordial but fascinating. He had heard I was a very good mother and was interested in how this reconciled with my public image.

At the time, I was going through a difficult stage of my life and was preoccupied with the problem of happiness in marriage. Naturally, the discussion turned to this theme—to marriage and the difficulties it faces in our society. I was fascinated to discover the wealth of insight he had into both the eternal and modern problems of love. He had a great ability to put his finger on the complexities of romantic life, concisely and simply. It was a surprise to me to discover a religious teacher who was so awake to the needs of intimacy between lovers, who understood that love must closely trace the contours of passion if it is to endure.

I was also intrigued to discover my beliefs about the importance of sensuality and sex in marriage being reflected back in fluent quotations from scripture. My father gave me a keen interest in mythology and folklore, and I have always had a huge respect for the wisdom buried in the mythologies of ancient cultures. So it was there—not in religious scripture—that I always looked to get perspective on human sexuality. On reflection, though, it is not surprising there is agreement between mythology and religion. Religious traditions are also human traditions, and sex and love are at the core of human experience. Such timeless and enduring expressions of human experience would naturally contain the same basic truths, the same delicate wisdom.

As fascinated as I was with his ideas, Rabbi Shmuley was also intrigued by mine. He was very interested in what he saw as apocalyptic contradictions in my character and how they related to the topics we were talking about. It was clear from our discussion that I—just like anyone—have experienced my share of heartache in life. But, he exclaimed, if anyone should be free of the loneliness of our society, surely, it should be me. It should be Pamela—the lifelong cover girl. The woman who—as the tabloids and gossip blogs would have it—could have any man she wants. If Pamela could be lonely, if her heart could be broken, that's an apocalypse! What hope is there for anyone else?

Of course, as we both knew, this is a myth—I am a human being just like anyone else. Experiences affect me as much as they do anyone else. And, as the great psychologist Carl Jung once wrote, "Even a happy life cannot be without a measure of darkness, and the word happy would lose its meaning if it were not balanced by sadness." But the question itself was fruitful. We decided that perhaps, instead of despair, it would give people hope or reprieve to know that we are all—without exception—on the great quest for romantic companionship and sexual contentment. During the course of our conversation, we realized that this supposed contradiction in me led deeper into the issues we were discussing, toward an understanding of the reasons for the death of love, of passion, of sex, in our contemporary society.

That was when we decided to work together on a book—a book that would capture these tensions, that would diagnose the problems of romantic passion in the twenty-first century, and that would point toward the solutions. Our book is a call for a fundamental change in relationships that will impact not only individuals but society as a whole. We want to inspire a revolution in human affairs that we believe must happen to afford the greatest possibility of romantic fulfillment to the greatest number of people. It is a sensual revolution that follows other cultural and sexual upheavals in our recent past, an adjustment that can restore balance to the way men and women relate to each other.

This transformation isn't something new to humanity. We experienced it a long time ago. We simply need to rediscover it and practice it once again in our modern relationships. Ancient mythologies carry its secrets. It is the first flowering of human sexuality in a time before histories were written, and it can be found throughout the literature and poetry and philosophy of every age and every culture. It is the enduring art of human intimacy.

Our book is about how it has been lost, and not for the first time. Human intimacy has been distorted before, by technologies that changed the way people connected to each other, and it was necessary each time for society to relearn how to love. In 1946, Nin wrote of "the dangerous time when mechanical voices, radios, telephones, take the place of human intimacies, and the concept of being in touch with millions brings a greater and greater poverty in intimacy and human vision."[3]

We are living through a similar change. How much has the "communications revolution" impoverished intimacy? There have been great strides forward in recent decades: sexual liberation, global activism, and a revolution in information. These are precious gains and should not be lost. But without a practiced understanding of the mysteries of human intimacy and sensuality, the technologies of our age can easily lead us into alienation, disaffection, and loneliness.

Shmuley and I agree: if the arts of intimacy and sensuality have been forgotten, they must be remembered again. Our culture must rediscover sensuality and sexiness, for the sake of meaning and value in our intimate lives. Our hope is that this book—the joint efforts of the most unlikely of co-authors: a rabbi and a *Playboy* cover girl—can help make that happen.

PREFACE BY

RABBI SHMULEY BOTEACH

When Pamela and I did our first TV interview together about sex and relationships on *The Dr. Oz Show*, Mehmet, our host and a friend of many years, asked me what she and I had in common that would cause us to share a joint message on eroticism and desire. I answered that it was all so plainly evident: An international sex symbol and a global object of desire, joining with a famous actress and animal rights activist, to rescue relationships.

The audience chuckled.

In truth, I had been offering a variation of this joke years before I ever met Pamela. When my book *Kosher Sex* was first published in the United Kingdom in 1998 and I began lecturing about the book around the world, people wanted to know what my credentials were to offer the public advice about sex. I responded, "My name is Shmu-ley, a contraction of two Hebrew root words. 'Shmu,' from the Hebrew root word, 'Shamoo,' meaning 'Killer Whale.' And 'Lee,' from the Hebrew root words 'Pamela Anderson Lee.' When you put them together, you get 'Larger than life Jewish sex god.'"

It's time for a more serious response. What could I, a rabbi, possibly have in common with one of the world's most recognizable sex symbols, enough to write an entire book about sensuality, eroticism, and relationships? The answer of course is being human. No matter our backgrounds or beliefs, we all essentially want the same thing, and that's especially true when it comes to relationships. What every person seeks in a romantic relationship is a contradiction: passion and intimacy, a lover who is also our soul mate, which is why it's so difficult to achieve.

On the one hand, we want passion and excitement—an end to boredom. We want to feel wild desire. We want someone's touch to take us to the moon and back in an erotic encounter. This comes from novelty, adventure, and risk. It comes from sharing our bodies with a lover. On the other hand, we seek companionship and an end to loneliness. We want true human warmth and authentic intimacy. This comes from precisely the opposite—sharing everyday experiences and routines with someone who begins as a stranger and ends up a soul mate.

Whether you're a rabbi or a *Playboy* cover girl, your desire for these conflicting needs is ever present. Being human entails searching for the fire of passion and the cool waters of intimacy. But fire and water don't mix. One extinguishes the other. Hence, most people fail at maximizing their relationships. We see this all around, especially when people say that their husband or wife is their best friend, connoting a close yet largely causal relationship bereft of erotic lust and fiery desire.

From our first conversations, Pamela and I agreed that every person pursues these opposing conditions and ends up frustrated. A celebrity of significant stature can feel this more acutely than most, as life lived on the red carpet can lead to an addiction to excitement. But the exclusivity of fame can induce a greater feeling of isolation and solitude.

I was amazed at Pamela's candor in discussing her own romantic journey and relationships. We hit it off from our first conversations on the subject. I am someone who values honesty and forthrightness, and Pamela was a model of trust and sharing. She has a world of experience with little hesitation to impart her valuable insights. It was clear that even if we disagreed somewhat on how a person might arrive at the twin goals of passion and intimacy, we were in full agreement that human fulfillment depends on reaching that destination.

Moreover, we agreed that the unique conditions of the modern world were undermining our ability to achieve these vital objectives. We agreed that porn was objectifying women and making it harder for men to experience feminine depth, even as we disagreed as to whether or not *Playboy* was a culprit. We agreed that the overtly sexual nature of modern society was impeding our experience of sensuality, even as we disagreed on what constituted sexual overexposure. And we agreed that lovemaking in our society had lost its erotic underpinnings, even as we disagreed on how it could be recaptured. Above all else, we agreed that what was needed to right this ship was not an evolutionary approach of predictable advice but a revolution in romantic thinking and erotic purpose. The result is a uniquely resplendent book, approached from utterly different experiences but pointing to the same promised land of passionate connection and intimate oneness.

The reader would be forgiven for assuming that in this book I, as the rabbi, am the traditionalist while Pamela represents the voice of liberal openness. In truth, Pamela wowed me from the outset with her solid commitment to traditional values. She spoke constantly of the inspiration she received from two parents who have loved each other in a decades-long marriage. I am the one who is a child of divorce. She told me of her deep desire to find fulfillment in a monogamous and committed relationship, while I was the one who wrote a book called *Kosher Adultery*, enjoining husbands and wives to have an affair with each other and spice up marriage with radical honesty and erotic fantasy. Above all else, Pamela shared with me her constant efforts to raise two young men who cherish and respect women, while I have strived, as the father of six daughters, to raise women who love marriage but never lose their independence. The moral of the story is that we humans are complicated creatures and what you see is not always what you get.

But then religion has been misunderstood as being hostile to sex from its inception. We've all heard the old wives' tales of priests warning boys that masturbation will lead to blindness or that Catholicism insists that sex is only for having babies. In truth, Judaism is a deeply erotic religion that orders a man to pleasure his wife sexually before he himself is pleasured. It is a religion that has long advocated that desire is more important than compatibility, that lust is greater than love, that carnal connection is the highest form of knowledge, and that sex is not for procreation but for conjoining husband and wife as bone of one bone and flesh of one flesh. The holiest book of the Jewish Biblical canon, says the Talmud, is Solomon's erotic love poem captured in Song of Solomon. In Judaism, sex is the very soul of marriage, and a termination of a couple's sex life constitutes a functional termination of the marriage itself. The pragmatic nature of marriage today as an institution primarily promoting companionship and friendship rather than fostering and sustaining deep erotic longing is utterly foreign to the Jewish faith.

Being a child of divorce forces you to address the confusing question of how two people responsible for your very existence could have ever been driven apart. Is there some sort of magic glue that can keep a man and woman happily under the same roof for the duration of their lives and can avoid that painful outcome, and what can you, their offspring, add to the equation? Is marriage an ossified institution that has passed its shelf life, and are your parents better off apart?

I was lucky in that, from an early age, I came down firmly on the side of marriage. I believe that having a soul mate as a lifelong partner is humanity's greatest blessing and that we have to find a remedy to the increasing landscape of broken hearts and shattered homes—and not just for the benefit of children who deserve to witness parents who are still in love, but for the participants in the marriage itself.

Marriage is not a prison. We do not stay together because kids need security or because we have a mortgage that has to be paid off. Rather, we stay together because desire and longing have been sustained and erotic interest in one another has increased through shared experienced. I reject marriage as an institution and embrace it instead as an instrument of erotic expression. I reject monogamy as deadening and embrace it instead as the avenue by which to fully focus our sexual lust. And I reject commitment as something confining and embrace it instead as the fullest means by which we humans attach ourselves to our other half.

As a student of Jewish mysticism, I have long been conditioned to identify the essence of another person from which all seemingly unrelated actions flow. Pamela is a fervent proponent of animal rights, and when we honored her at our Champions of Jewish Values International Awards Gala for standing up for Israel, she praised the Jewish state as a country with one of the highest rates of vegetarianism and veganism (wow, who knew?). I have since come to understand that her unmatched championing of animal welfare stems from her deep attachment to every incarnation of life. And what is sexuality other than humankind's most passionate expression of feeling alive? It is this feeling that we wish to impart to the reader.

In our time, the deep yearning for sexual connection is being replaced with a shallow desire for sexual conquest. Building erotic yearning is being replaced with immediately satiating every sexual itch. And sexuality is overtaking sensuality. The two are not the same. Whereas the former is a strictly carnal experience of bodily friction leading to climax, the latter is an electrifying elixir of psychological and spiritual indulgence leading to the orchestration of two halves as one whole. The former employs our genitalia as the principal sexual organ, while the latter melds the mind and heart into an explosive carnival of sensual delight.

Should we be surprised, then, that ours is a generation of marital sexual famine, where the average couple has sex once a week for seven minutes on average, and nearly one out of four couples has no sex at all? When sex is reduced to unimaginative predictability and rote, when lovemaking becomes a rushed means to orgasmic end, when foreplay is passed over for immediate penetration, should we be surprised that television becomes the most exciting thing happening in the bedroom?

Our book seeks to reverse these corrosive trends by restoring lovemaking to what it was always meant to be: a deep and passionate desire to know and experience another person in the deepest possible way. It may seem odd that two bodies locked together in an erotic charge can provide for a far deeper understanding than a conversation or the exchange of ideas. But then, knowing someone experientially is always superior to knowing the person intellectually. The heart has always been superior to the mind. That we are blind to this truth speaks volumes about the blissful ignorance of relationships and how much sex has been degraded in our time.

And that's what so intrigued me about Pamela. While she was being portrayed as the object of fantasy and the incarnation of desire, she was herself fantasizing about passionate monogamy and an erotic connection in a committed relationship.

This is not a book for the faint of heart. It rejects prudery in favor of erotic openness just as it rejects sexual license in favor of romantic focus. The false choice that has been visited upon us moderns between the extremes of a pragmatic and predictable partnership, on the one hand, and base pornography on the other is one that should be repudiated utterly.

It's time we recaptured the ancient idea of the sacred feminine not as a woman of wifely duty and pious virtue but as a risk-taking adventuress whose very being captures the infinite possibility of joyous sex. Husbands must come to recognize that even the most devoted wife can never be fully possessed. Her sexuality is an overflowing fountain, her erotic needs a bottomless pit, her carnal desire an ever-expansive plain.

That men no longer see their wives this way is one of the reasons they turn to shallow substitutes like porn, which dulls their senses and makes a mockery of true erotic imagination. The sensual woman is a walking magnet, always pulling the masculine presence even as she gravitates toward one man who becomes her chosen.

If it's true that our troubled world—filled with so much friction and strife—needs to "make love, not war," then it's equally true that love

Sarasota County
Public Libraries

www.scgov.net/library
941-861-1100

Number of items:

1

Barcode:31969025898924
Title:Lust for love : rekindling intimacy and
passion in your relationship / Pamela
Anderson and Rabbi Shm
Due:4/5/2019

3/15/2019   4:38 PM

cannot be made when we are constantly fighting an inner war. The battle for sexual focus—to be passionate and intimate about one person—is one we must finally engage in, freeing ourselves to experience the blessings of erotic liberation.

Pamela and I are two distinct people, but in this book, we have found one voice. A voice that calls for love and appreciation. A voice that calls for desire and passion. A voice that calls for commitment and dedication. A voice that calls for erotic attachment and sensual connection. And a voice that calls for a new relationship between the masculine and feminine.

Happy reading.

Part One

HAVE WE FORGOTTEN HOW TO MAKE LOVE?

CHAPTER 1

The Art of Intimacy

This art of love discloses the special and sacred identity of the other person. Love is the only light that can truly read the secret signature of the other person's individuality and soul. Love alone is literate in the world of origin; it can decipher identity and destiny.

JOHN O'DONOHUE

O scar Wilde once wrote, "One should always be in love. That is the reason one should never marry." We believe he's wrong. We believe intimacy isn't lost in marriage. We believe passionate, romantic love can exist within a long-term relationship, lasting years after the echoes of wedding bells fade. We reject the belief that we have to put off marriage or reject monogamy altogether to have exciting, passionate, toe-curling sex.

The notion of marriage being the death of Eros is one that is foreign to our thinking. Marriage is where sex flourishes—or at least it should. The real death of sex is caused by a culture that has rejected the foundations of intimacy that fuel passion—emotional and spiritual connection, subjective knowledge of another human being, and sexual restraint that builds anticipation—choosing instead mechanical detachment, objectification, and immediate gratification.

Pamela

One of my favorite writers, essayist Anaïs Nin, once said people don't know how to make love, to discover the artistry of intimacy, because in their "microscopic examination of sexual activity" *they exclude important aspects of intimacy that are the necessary fuel to ignite it.* "This is what gives sex its surprising textures, its subtle transformations, its aphrodisiac elements," *she writes. When you don't have it,* "you are shrinking your world of sensations. You are withering it, starving it, draining its blood." *Instead, we need to find the source of sexual power, which is curiosity and passion. When you don't nourish it,* "you're watching its little flame die of asphyxiation. Sex does not thrive on monotony."[1] *Sex can't survive without passion and intimacy.*

An erotic relationship flourishes when there's curiosity and familiarity, passion and emotional connection, fantasy and realism. A key way to hold these apparent contradictions together is by practicing the principles of eroticism: unavailability, mystery, forbiddenness, and vertical discovery. When these are woven into a relationship, a vibrant life full of passion and intimacy is the result.

Overfamiliarity can kill passion, but this can be avoided by putting some healthy distance into the relationship. Unavailability generates frustrated desire—that hunger you feel when you're first getting to know each other. You long for your lover's kiss, to see his body, to discover how he feels against you, but you can't always have him. He's just beyond your reach. It might seem like unavailability would be impossible in a marriage, but it isn't. That hunger you once felt can be experienced again and again.

Mystery injects a sense of curiosity and novelty into the relationship.

You don't know everything about this person you've fallen in love with; there's still so much to discover, something new and amazing. You always want to know more about him, but he's not easily understood or readily available. He remains a mystery to unravel. This attracts you, keeping your interest alive.

In the same way, forbiddenness adds another layer of excitement by injecting a little naughtiness into the relationship. Let's admit it, sin is exciting. Wanting something you can't have gets your heart beating, your skin flushed, your mind racing. This fuels passion. Marriage seems to close the door on this possibility because it's completely legal— there's nothing forbidden about marriage, nothing sinful. But this element can still be injected into the relationship in little ways that feed eroticism.

The final principle—vertical discovery—is essential to both intimacy and passion. Vertical renewal is when we plumb the depths of another, taking the time to know them, discovering what they really like, learning new interests and passions, getting to know them at deeper and deeper levels as we explore their body and mind. We become bored with one another when we think we know all there is to know, but human beings are multifaceted, especially if we develop ourselves individually to become more interesting and to experience more of life. The person you're married to should never become a bore, and they won't if you both take the time to discover new and wondrous things about each other. Penetrate those depths. Peel back the layers. This can be deeply erotic and inflame passion as you lead one another down new paths, share new insights, and learn new perspectives. This lust for knowledge, for understanding, for life is a lust for love when shared by two people who intimately and continually discover each other.

Living a life of passionate connectedness is not theoretical. We've seen it. We've experienced the joy of it. We've met couples who embody these principles.

RABBI SHMULEY

I have counseled many men and women and have known a couple
for years who live according to these principles. Their marriage is a
shining example of lasting love and intimacy. Mike and Sue's relationship is based on total honesty. They have a sensual and sexual
openness that they've worked on for many years. They can have
erotic conversations with each other about fantasy, sexual desire,
and sensual needs without conflict because they've pushed beyond
inhibitions.

You would think this would be natural for a married couple, but
it isn't. Many couples live closed off from each other, often afraid to
be vulnerable with the other, sexually and emotionally. This erodes
passion and love over time. Mike and Sue have overcome those
fears even to the point that Mike can listen to his wife's fantasies
about him and others without getting hurt. He learns from her so
he can be a better lover and husband. He sees this sharing as an
expansion of his wife's desire. He admits it's slightly threatening to
him, but he can get past it because he knows her honesty makes
them closer.

Even after several years of marriage, their sex life is strong and
sensual. They don't do a lot of quickies, but spend time with each
other, seeking vertical renewal. Sue doesn't exist to satisfy Mike's
urges. They engage in kissing and giving each other massages.
This doesn't always lead to intercourse; sometimes just touching
is enough. In fact, delayed gratification makes things much more
exciting to them, and they have no problem stoking the fires
of desire and saving the best parts for later. There's a romantic
build-up that connects them through sensuality, sound, scent, and
touch.

Sex is important in their relationship, but it isn't everything, of
course. It's not the apex of their relationship. They also engage in

constant romantic activity, not mushy things like buying flowers and gifts. Their romance is integrated into their daily lives because they're about being, not just doing. They know how to be present with each other, sharing their thoughts and feelings throughout the day, taking walks, and having a sense of oneness in everything they do. They haven't lost their sense of individuality, but they are two people who comprise a larger whole because they share their hopes and dreams. They laugh a lot, and when they hurt each other they ask for forgiveness. When they've inflicted pain, they acknowledge it; they don't deny or ignore it. They heal the wound and bridge the gap that has been created by their own thoughtlessness. This keeps bitterness from building. They don't have to be burdened with constantly educating each other about what hurts them. They see it on their own, and they fix it.

They're also very loving parents. Their love isn't exclusive, focused only on them. It's shared. Friendship is important, and children are important. They know the balance of being parents and a couple. A loving, erotic relationship doesn't mean they need to cut themselves off from the world. They stay communally engaged, and this enriches their relationship because it stimulates and improves them as individuals. They don't live in isolation from the world, their children, or each other. These intimate connections and their intersections in their lives make their relationship vibrant, full of life and love.

When Mike and Sue are together, there is a deep respect between them. Sue is a very feminine woman, and there's a quiet dignity to her. She can command the conversation at the table with a certain feminine subtlety. It's obvious that there's so much depth to her, and Mike finds her endlessly interesting. He feels privileged to be with a woman as developed as she is. There is an ease of comfort between them. It's not forced, and it's not showy. It's small gestures. He defers to her and is a little in awe of her. She never engages in emasculation toward him. No little digs directed his way. Certainly no eye rolling. She respects him and believes she is married to a good man. She tells him this constantly. This mutual respect enhances their love.

More than anything else, their relationship is a blessing to others. Their friends and extended family are blessed, and their children are blessed, because they too want to get married just like their parents. They want to have the kind of intimate relationship their parents have. They don't want just cheap, unimaginative sex. They want lifelong partners. They see that their parents' marriage is passionate and intimate, and they want the same.

This is the kind of relationship many people want but don't have. They want that intimate connection with passionate sex. They want a full life shared with the one person who completes them. Some have experienced it briefly, but they haven't been able to sustain it, and its memory hangs in their heart forever as they long for more than just a familiar face sleeping on the other side of the bed.

Pamela

I've also experienced this kind of relationship, and know how satisfying and enriching it is. It was a special bond I will always treasure. There were other romances before that, but none compared with that relationship. In those other relationships, there was room for self-consciousness and doubt. I'd ask, "Is this love?" and not really know the answer. This relationship was different. There were no doubts, no reservations, no second-guessing. The two of us were more comfortable with each other than on our own. Everything flowed from an immediate mutual recognition, a sense of being in step, not just physically but psychologically too.

Everything felt as if it had been lined up perfectly: our sense of humor, our rhythms, our sudden passion for each other, our easy exchange of affection and warmth. Maybe this is why poets compare love to the alignment of stars. He knew, without knowing, how to complement me, how to make me feel safe and happy with myself, and I knew how to do the same for him. It was like a dance that had taken off, suddenly no longer merely following the steps or going through the motions, but now a force of its own that felt right and natural.

I realized that all that had come before had been learning the steps for this relationship. And I also knew that, like a dance, it was something that required commitment from both of us, something we would need to maintain together if it was to continue.

Not all such relationships last, and often the loss of love like this is part of the learning experience too. But when I hear people express skepticism about the possibility of real love in the twenty-first century, I remember that love and how it was once just right, and I know: it is possible. More than that, it's necessary.

CHAPTER 2

Our Deep Need

Love is the only sane and satisfactory answer to the problem of human existence.

ERICH FROMM

When it comes to love, we want it all: love and romance, intimacy and passion, mystery and familiarity, fusion and freedom. But today it seems like fewer people are actually getting it. They find themselves in a sexual wasteland, often alone or disconnected from the one they're with—they're together, sharing the same space, but they're essentially apart, because there's no intimacy, no fire that burns between them, no passion that quickens their bodies and their hearts.

Both of us, in our different spheres, have heard too many accounts from people who are struggling in lifeless relationships, and the stories are heartbreaking. They feel neglected, alone, and incomplete. They have sex, but it's like sleeping with a ghost. Their partners are distant. The sex they have is joyless and automatic, or they're not having sex at all—even in marriage.

Pamela

Rabbi Shmuley has seen this trend over thirty years of counseling, and I've seen it too, throughout my career—women telling me their lonely stories, often with tears in their eyes as they pour out their hearts, sharing their most private anxieties and fears.

I don't know why they feel so free to talk to me about their feelings and desires, but they do. Maybe it's my public image, which has always had a life of its own. Ever since my first photo shoot for Playboy, *sex has been a part of my image. Perhaps they sense from this that I will understand. I won't judge.*

RABBI SHMULEY

I've experienced the same thing in a different way—people who are willing, even desperate, to divulge their deepest needs to me. You would think they wouldn't tell a religious figure about their hunger for sex and intimacy. But they do, because they are desperate for answers and guidance in their relationships. Sexual desire is a natural part of who we are. It's a yearning inside of us that needs to be met through healthy expression and not ignored.

Whatever the reason people share, we don't question it. We listen while they tell us their lonely secrets. "He hasn't touched me in months," we hear from women. "I'm waiting upstairs in lingerie, and he's in the basement staring at a computer screen. I'm real; I'm flesh and blood. But he is lost in a fantasy world. It doesn't have to be this way, but I don't know how to change it." Others are unhappy even with many lovers. They have plenty of sex, but something is missing. "I feel more isolated than ever," they say. "I feel less human, as if I'm a cog in a machine. I wait for Prince Charming, but he never comes."

Pamela

I can relate to how they feel. This astonishes most people because they assume I'm above it all. If anyone has escaped this kind of loneliness, they think, it must be me. I haven't though; I know exactly what they're feeling. I too have experienced the sorrows, and joys, of love. I know what it's like to go to sleep beside the person you love while feeling as if an ocean lies between you. I know how at this "unique distance from isolation," *as Philip Larkin wrote in his poem* "Talking in Bed," "It becomes still more difficult to find/ Words at once true and kind/Or not untrue and not unkind."[1]

And I've seen the other side of it too. I've had passionate but disappointing sex that was without meaning or possibility. I've seen how a hookup culture arrests our emotional development and makes us unable to love. I've looked into the hedonistic playground of modern courtship and seen emptiness.

This is why I have so much compassion for both men and women suffering these dislocations of our age—I know firsthand their pain and heartache.

Neither of us believes these are stories from a few lonely women and men. The emotional pain they report goes deeper and is suffered more widely than they realize. It is the common experience of love in the twenty-first century. Something is happening to the way we relate to each other. Sex is being made more transactional, and love is being starved of passion. These stories point to something bigger and more troubling than individual heartache: the retreat of Eros from human relationships. This is a widespread cultural problem, and we can't address the broader crisis if we don't understand it and how we all share in it.

We want to help people understand how we got here. We want them to find happiness in their relationships and their marriages, to rediscover selfless sensuality, caring, letting go, and giving with wild abandon. We want people to more easily achieve the deep and peaceful joys of being loved and desired. We want to persuade them not to deny their pain because they think alienation is somehow normal or right. By bringing together our very different experiences, we can put a name to this crisis and begin to address it: Sex—good sex that is adventurous and meaningful, engaging the mind and body, held afloat by love and desire—is dying in America, but it's not too late to save it. The solutions are there if we only know where to look. The art of intimacy and passion can be rediscovered.

So many problems in relationships today can be traced to the bedroom. Couples let everyday worries and the routine of marriage disrupt the very thing that is essential to maintaining their marital bond. They're often not even aware it's happening. They just see the effects and wonder about the cause.

RABBI SHMULEY

This was the case for a couple I counseled who had been married for eleven years. All the passion had been drained from their relationship, even though they didn't realize it at first. They just knew something was missing. The wife, in particular, was unhappy. They were in their mid-thirties, young and attractive, and they initially came for counseling because the husband never wanted to be home. He didn't put it that way, but the wife felt like he was avoiding her.

As they started to break down some of the problems in the marriage, I asked them about their sex life. They said it was very good. When I asked how often they had sex, they said about once every three weeks for about twenty minutes. They said it matter-of-factly, but the fact is their sex life wasn't "very good"—and that was one of the main problems. How do you expect to maintain intimacy, make a woman feel desired, and give her the attention she craves if you're only making love to her about once a month for a mere twenty minutes? The husband's excuse was fatigue; he was just too tired when he came home from work. But with that statement, he thoughtlessly diminished his wife's sensual needs. He was neglecting a part of her that was longing to be fed and nourished. This deprivation led to tremendous dissatisfaction in the marriage.

Eighty to ninety percent of the people who come to me for counseling are just like this couple; they're barely touching each other. They don't say that up front, but when pressed, they admit it. They often think this is normal, but it's not. It's like forgetting how to do something as natural as drinking water. When a married couple goes weeks or months without having sex, something's wrong.

The reason many couples don't realize it's a problem is because there's such a diminished expectation of sex today. They see it as a bonus, something that happens after all the really "important" things are done. Taking care of kids. Paying bills. Cleaning the house. Shopping for groceries. Answering the boss's latest text. Watching television. Scanning Twitter. Posting pics on Facebook. Sex comes last. It's a luxury, not a necessity. It's icing on the cake. They fail to see that it's so much more, that it's foundational to everything else. It's not just the icing or even the cake, it's the heat that turns the batter into something you can sink your teeth into, something that will feed your soul and your relationship.

If couples want to save their marriage, they can't ignore the importance of sex. While they might think the spontaneous, electrifying sex they once enjoyed is no longer necessary because their relationship has morphed into something deeper, this is a delusion. They still need that spark, that fire, but too often they don't get it because men don't want to take the time to keep the fire burning, to blow on the embers and stoke the flames. They don't want to spend time investing in intimacy. Everything has become secondary to immediate gratification. Consumption has replaced connection. Men have been trained out of taking the time to give a woman what she desires—and what she desires is to be desired. This is true for a woman when she's being chased, and it's true even after she's been caught.

This problem cuts both ways, of course. Some women are failing—and sometimes outright refusing—to meet their partner's sexual needs.

RABBI SHMULEY

This was true for a couple I counseled who knew their relationship lacked intimacy, but they didn't know why or how to fix it. The wife felt like her husband didn't pay enough attention to her, but every time he tried to touch her, she would recoil. He would try again the next night, but she just wasn't interested. The husband complained that he had tried everything to bring life to their marriage, to make it more erotic—lighting candles, buying her lingerie, and creating a romantic atmosphere—but she would always turn him down. Every time.

The wife didn't see how she was part of the problem. She failed to understand how emasculating it is for a man to try to make love to his wife and be rejected every single night. In a moment of frustration during counseling, the husband said to her, *"You have utterly deprived me; you have starved my basic needs as a man."* She snapped back: *"That's exactly right; it's all about your needs as a man. It's never about me as a woman."*

At this point, I said to her, "I understand that you feel distant, and that you don't want to share your body with someone you think has not been loving, and that sex can't be like a light switch you can just flick on and off. But why are you assuming the desire for sex is only about him? Let's say he made the mistake of only trying to turn you on at night and not during the day, and sex was his way of trying to connect instead of doing it through communication, appreciation, and compliments. Let's say he failed to approach you holistically, that he was only focused on the sexual aspect. Why are you assuming that effort was fraudulent and that it was all about him? Yes, his approach was wrong. But that doesn't mean it was insincere. Is it possible that this is a form of payback on your part—that if he's going to deprive you of sharing emotionally, then you're going to deprive him of intimacy?"

She admitted that was exactly the case. Her husband made her feel unfeminine and undesirable, and she was making him suffer because rejecting him would strike him in the most personal way. She was right; it was very hurtful. And her husband was clueless about how women don't respond to men who want physical intimacy in place of emotional connectedness. But she wasn't helping the situation at all. Sex shouldn't be used as a weapon or a form of punishment. Sex is a bridge to connect two people, and sometimes you need to rekindle the spark in the relationship using the nuclear option, and sex is that nuclear option because it involves the strongest emotions we have. If you want intimacy in a committed relationship, making love is one of the ways to get it. It's the doorway that opens one soul to another.

When a man feels distant from a woman, he wants to feel immediately close, so he bridges that distance the best way he knows how—with sex. If real connection is ignored, however, taking this "short-cut" to intimacy is misguided. It doesn't work because the woman might be put off by it, as we saw in the case above. But that doesn't make the *desire* insincere. It's what the husband thinks will bring him closer to his wife. But this is only true if *making love* overtakes *having sex*. Lovemaking is foundational in a relationship. It should be done with emotional investment and manifest itself in tactility and touch.

In Judaism, using sex as a selfish end in itself or as a weapon is strictly forbidden because the purpose of sex is to reinforce the marital bond. Sex isn't considered just a man's basic need. It's also a woman's basic need, and more importantly, it's the couple's basic need, because marriage is two people made one—and sex is integral to creating that oneness, not just physically but emotionally. Husbands and wives must understand the centrality of sex to a healthy marriage and never allow the passion to be lost through neglect.

This is taken very seriously in the Jewish religion. A husband or wife can sue for divorce if either withholds sex as unwarranted punishment, just as a couple can be divorced if a man refuses to make love to his wife or neglect her carnal and emotional needs. He can't just use her for his own gratification—he must please her as well. Sex is not seen as a "selfish indulgence" that can be denied for any reason or used without thought to the other person's needs. It's foundational to the marriage. A functional termination of the sexual dimension of marriage is treated as a functional termination of the marriage itself. It undermines the relationship and erodes the marital bond.

Even if you're not Jewish, there's much wisdom to be learned from this. If both the man and the woman see sex as essential to the marriage, they will value it. They will cherish it, even in times of conflict. When they're feeling distant, hurt, and ignored, this is the time to nurture their intimate bond, not neglect it.

CHAPTER 3

A Sexual Famine

Terrifying, that the loss of intimacy with one person results in the freezing over of the world, and the loss of oneself.

JAMES BALDWIN

There must be a change in our culture's attitude toward sex. It's time for couples to bring sensuality, intensity, and desire back into their relationships. Men and women need to be desired, they need the lustful attention of their partner—they crave it. It's natural, and both are hurting when they don't get it. It fulfills them like nothing else, chasing away the specter of loneliness that hovers over us all. A woman needs her partner's touch, his breath on her skin, his hungry kisses, his eyes fixed only on her. She needs his companionship and his desire, just as he needs hers. Human beings are not meant to be isolated. "The deepest need of man," as the philosopher Erich Fromm wrote, "is the need to overcome his separateness, to leave the prison of his aloneness."[1] It's right there in the Bible, at the beginning of Genesis, when the first thing God declares is, "It's not good for humans to be alone." Men and women need passionate, desirous love.

Instead of getting it, women are either denying their needs or they're trying to compete with entertainment, distraction, and pornography. Too many men are looking for self-worth by accumulating assets or power, binging on sports, or becoming lost in a joyless addiction to pornography. They have forgotten their partners as a source of self-worth—either because they've substituted a superficial distraction for them or because, out of loneliness, they venture online looking for a quick fix. When you think about it, films and photographs of other people having sex can't fill the emptiness they feel. Porn is just a simulation of the real thing, and it has no sexiness of its own—all of its eroticism is borrowed from the need to be intimate with someone else in a deeply sensual way.

There's nothing sensual about pornography, no connection, no intimacy. It's cold and mechanical, and it's desensitizing us, making us more machine-like and emotionally impaired. Anaïs Nin captures this sentiment well in *Delta of Venus* when she writes, "Sex loses all its power and magic when it becomes explicit, mechanical, overdone, when it becomes a mechanistic obsession. It becomes a bore." It's wrong "not to mix it with emotion, hunger, desire, lust, whims, caprices, personal ties, deeper relationships that change its color, flavor, rhythms, intensities."[2] It's wrong to let it die.

This sexual famine is not only disrupting marriages, it's also causing depression and loss of self-worth. In a snapshot of this problem, a study of more than 700 South African women by an antidepressant pharmaceutical company found that 70 percent of the women surveyed said lack of sexual intimacy in their relationships made them feel depressed.[3] Despite eight in ten of the women describing their sex drive as healthy, 15 percent cited their partner's lack of interest as one of the main reasons they're not having sex as often as they'd like. "As many as 64% measured their self-esteem, femininity and desirability directly to how their partner responds to them sexually."[4] This doesn't mean these women are weak or overly reliant on a man. It does mean that there is an interdependency that we all experience and that we seek validation in the arms of the person pledged to us. Seeking tactility and the affirmation of loving touch does not make us weak, but human. It makes us natural, healthy men and women who desire completion and companionship with one another. Women and men need that physical—and spiritual—connection. Without it, they can become depressed and lonely.

Of course, not everyone needs a companion to be whole. We're well aware of the famous feminist declaration that "a woman needs a man the way a fish needs a bicycle." This is taking things way too far, but we recognize that men and women can lead productive, purposeful lives as individuals and not just in relationships. But how much better is it when we *can* live life in love rather than alone? How much better is it when love makes life easier rather than imposing an emotional burden? When we're surrounded by love, everything becomes more colorful, more beautiful, and suffused with more meaning.

People look for love because they feel alive when another desires them—when they're *known*. For most people, when there's no intimacy, no sex, it's like they're living in a desert, where they become thirsty and miserable. This is no way to live, suffering in quiet misery. And it's actually worse when you're in a relationship and you're neglected. A poll of 3,000 couples from a dating site in Great Britain bears this out. The poll found that most people are unhappy in their relationship because the sexual fire is burning low or has gone out completely.[5] More than six out of ten adults surveyed said they need to improve their sex lives, and four out of ten have thought about getting a divorce. Couples admitted "lack of sex, spontaneity, affection and romance makes it hard to maintain a loving relationship."[6] And more than half said "their partner was no longer the 'affectionate and giving' person they were when they first started dating."[7] Half of the people polled were hopeless this could change.[8] They're stuck in a rut and don't know how to reignite the passion they once had for each other. So they settle in, accept the death of Eros as the norm and force themselves to be satisfied with a platonic relationship, or they ditch the effort and go looking for passion elsewhere, either by cheating or leaving.

The truth is, marriage isn't based on platonic love. It can't thrive that way. This doesn't mean you should always be swinging from the chandeliers, but a fervent desire for one another needs to be alive and well. This is what makes marriage unique. This is why people choose to get married—for erotic love—and Eros is inseparable from lust and desire. Husbands and wives aren't supposed to be merely best friends or roommates. They're supposed to be passionate for each other and filled with sexual longing, drinking from each other's fountain—as the Bible describes it—intoxicated by their love.[9] This is what makes a partnership formed around sexual union different from every other relationship.

If marriage were supposed to be just about unconditional love, a woman would never leave her parents' house. Why would she? Who loves her better, or more unconditionally, than her parents? Not only does she eventually leave, when she's fifteen she has to be positively coerced into staying home. As she matures and becomes a woman, the omnipotence of her parents' love suddenly becomes impotent. Amazingly, she craves the love of a stranger. Then she falls in love and marries a man she's attracted to sexually, and he's attracted to her. They're not just friends—they lust after each other with erotic love. "Bone of one bone and flesh of one flesh" is not something friends experience. Buddies at the bar don't share that deep, committed intimacy. Best friends aren't driven by lustful hunger to consume each other. If they are, they're no longer simply best friends. They're lovers, and they've developed a different kind of relationship—an erotic one.

Too many marriages today are settling into a boring friendship mode. A report in *Newsweek* estimates that "15 to 20 percent of couples have sex no more than 10 times a year, which is how the experts define sexless marriage."[10] Other studies have found that 4.9 percent of married men and 6.5 percent of married women between the ages of nineteen and fifty-nine say they haven't had sex in the past year.[11] This is an increase from the mid-1990s, when researchers found that only 1.3 percent of married men and 2.6 percent of married women hadn't had sex in a year.[12]

One of the reasons cited for the decrease in sexual activity is "habituation": "While sex may be exciting at first, over time one becomes accustomed to sex with a spouse, until eventually what once was exciting is now rather dull."[13] The reasons for this lack of interest are complex—age, declining health, decrease in libido, the loss of imagination, and a failure to face up to and work through emotional differences. Regardless of the reasons, this dearth of sex in marriage has negative consequences because couples who are sexually inactive are more likely to get divorced than those who are having sex. Couples who remain sexually active stay married longer, and these couples actually have sex more often than those who are the same age and recently married.[14]

Other researchers have seen the same trends. Jean Twenge and colleagues published a paper in *Archives of Sexual Behavior* that examined declines in sexual frequency among American adults from 1989 to 2014 and found a steady decline in adults having sex during those years with a dramatic downturn after 2000.[15] Since the 1990s, American adults have been having sex nine fewer times every year.[16] This is attributed to more people not getting married (unmarried people typically have less sex than married couples) and married or partnered people having less sex.[17] Twenge's group found that sexual frequency among partnered people has been on the decline, whereas it has remained steady among those who aren't married.[18] This is a stunning trend since one of the advantages to being married has always been greater frequency of sex.

Researchers say people aren't having as much sex because of jobs, longer workdays, childcare, medications that reduce the sex drive, and a pervasive preoccupation with entertainment and social media, including pornography in isolation.[19] But these aren't the *root* cause. It's something much more fundamental. *Why* do couples choose to put work, children, entertainment, and porn before having sex, despite the fact that frequency of sex in marriage is associated with a greater sense of well-being?[20] It's because they've lost the very thing that makes their relationship unique, the one thing that brought them together in the first place: desire. They've allowed lust to die.

As a result, they're not as happy as they could be, and with so many people miserable in their relationships,[21] no wonder the United States has dropped from the third happiest nation in the world in 2007 to nineteenth in 2016—and this could be one reason.[22] The problem isn't marriage itself, but a loss of desire—the fire that keeps the marriage alive. Instead of finding connection, intimacy, and fulfillment in the bedroom with the person they love, they're busy doing other things or they're online frittering away days and nights in a detached, artificial world. Spending time in virtual reality might be fun for kids, but researchers have found that adults over thirty are becoming less happy—and one of the reasons cited is they spend too much time on social media.[23] They're seeking companionship in entertainment and Internet chat rooms instead of with their spouse. They're texting instead of talking, creating a greater divide.[24] They're living in the same house, together but alone.

There was a time when marriage offered a respite from the toils of the world, where a couple could come together as one flesh, exploring each other's bodies in the security and familiarity of erotic love. One of the great things about getting married was, "We can have sex any time we want!" Sex in marriage was like drinking wine and eating honey from a honeycomb—a beautiful description from the Song of Solomon.[25] It was something to be celebrated and enjoyed. Now, marriage has become a sexless drudgery. No wonder young people are putting off marriage until they're older. Back in 1960, at the cusp of the sexual revolution, 72 percent of Americans eighteen and over were married, with the median age for a first marriage being twenty years for women and twenty-three for men.[26] Now, only about half of them are tying the knot,[27] with the median age for a first marriage reaching its highest point in 2016: 29.5 years for men and 27.4 for women.[28]

There are a number of reasons for this, including sex outside of marriage, economics, and women in the workforce. The economic pressures
of the twenty-first century mean fewer people can afford to tie the knot
and settle down as early in life as previous generations. Rising house prices
and the cost of raising children mean fewer people opt for that kind of
financial commitment. And for those more fortunate, why settle when you
can wait, find the perfect man, and marry for love, not financial dependence? That's the number one reason 88 percent of Americans want to get
married anyway: for love.[29]

But love is shriveling on the vine because its highest expression, namely,
making love, is dying, causing marriage to be unattractive. Instead of sweet
wine, it's turning to vinegar. The blazing fire is going cold, leaving couples
poking among the ashes for a spark to reignite their marriage. Too often
they're looking for the wrong solutions. They're missing the very thing
that is fundamental to a successful marriage. They've forgotten how to
enjoy sensual sex, the teasing, touching, breathing, building, connecting,
and exploding that melts into a long, blissful embrace. They've forgotten
how to lust for love.

CHAPTER 4

Failure of the Sexual Revolution

A key feature of sexual revolution is the large-scale publication and commercialization of details that were once secret. Sexuality has been trivialized. The interesting thing about this is that exaggerated portrayals apparently destroy desire more effectively than any repression.

VOLKMAR SIGUSCH

The decline of sex in the twenty-first century is surprising since the sexual revolution of the 1960s was all about making sex more free and enjoyable, especially for women. For too long, sex was primarily for procreation. Sexual imagination was considered inimical to piety and religious observance. Strange as it sounds, in sanitizing sex it was actually becoming disconnected from its Biblical origin. The Bible is clear: Sex is not primarily about procreation or even performing some marital duty. Rather, it's about joining two people to become one flesh. "Therefore shall a man leave his father and his mother, and shall cleave unto his wife: and they shall be one flesh."[1] The purpose of sex is intimacy. Let the evolutionary scientists say what they want, sex is not principally about making babies. Nor is it only about propagating our genes. Rather, it's about truly knowing another person. Sex enlivens life with intense emotion and intimacy. One only has to turn to the pages of Song of Solomon to find the Bible's celebration of sex for the sheer glory of it:

> Your lips are like a scarlet ribbon;
>   your mouth is lovely.
> Your temples behind your veil
>   are like the halves of a pomegranate.
> Your neck is like the tower of David,
>   built with courses of stone;
>   on it hang a thousand shields,
>   all of them shields of warriors.
> Your breasts are like two fawns,
>   like twin fawns of a gazelle
>   that browse among the lilies.
> Until the day breaks
>   and the shadows flee,
> I will go to the mountain of myrrh
>   and to the hill of incense.
> You are altogether beautiful, my darling;
>   there is no flaw in you.[2]

This concept of sex and women's sexuality has ebbed and flowed throughout human history and across cultures, with periods of sexual oppression followed by liberating movements, one reaction to another. We passed through the sweeping romances of the ancient world to the darkness and chivalry of medieval times, the legalistic dogma of thirteenth- and sixteenth-century Europe to the sexual tolerance and loose morals of the French court, all the way to the Victorian era's severe morality and strict social conventions. During this "age of innocence," sex developed a somber overtone with its focus on procreation. Gone was the vitality and sensuality of sex sporadically known in other times. The Victorian era anesthetized it, except in the underbelly of society where upper-class men stripped off their finely pressed clothes and slept with prostitutes. Society looked the other way, of course. But women received no latitude. Enjoyment of sex by a woman was considered unseemly, and any public display of her sexuality earned her the label of whore or prostitute. Even her genitalia were reduced to being called a purse—a functional description where a man spends both his money and his sexual urges.

The sexual revolution ripped that social fabric to shreds. Women rejected the repressive Victorian conventions and codes of conduct that lingered into the 1950s. They broke the chains of a patriarchal culture that made them feel ashamed of their sexual appetites and locked them into social responsibilities deemed appropriate for their "softer" natures. Gender roles were challenged and redefined, as women left traditional roles to become entrepreneurs, politicians, doctors, and lawyers. With the legalization of contraceptives for unmarried couples, IUDs, the pill, and legal abortion, sex became unmoored from procreation. Women—and sex along with it—were released from their Victorian cage of functionality to explore, experiment, and express. In a word, sex became natural again, infused with creativity, excitement, and freedom. Female sexuality was unleashed. As a *Playboy* playmate, Pamela participated in that liberation of female sexuality—the application of the principles of free expression to the sexual expression of women. We might disagree on whether *Playboy* is genuinely liberating or whether there is an exploitative side to it, but there can be no denying that *Playboy* gained immense popularity as a rebellion against sexual repression.

But something went wrong. From those first promising days through the age of the Internet, sex became overexposed and cheapened. It became an end in itself. In our society's quest to liberate sex, we lost the meaning of sex, the sensuality of sex, and the fundamental purpose of sex—to bring two people together and make them one, body and soul. The authentic, emotional, connected dimension was lost. It became solely about the physical, and the spiritual was abandoned. It became about self-gratification instead of other-gratification. The thrill of the chase gave way to the thrill of being thrilled, and like drug addicts, we now need more to get our high. Something new. Something different. Something extreme. It's not enough simply to make love to one person, discovering who they are and what they enjoy, learning how their body responds and what brings them the most pleasure. Instead, we have sex with one person after another, ordering them on dating apps like a pizza, watching pornography, resorting to masochism, violence, and even cruelty.

We've abandoned sensuality, becoming uncomfortably numb. Men have to take drugs at a younger age just to get an erection because they're desensitized, bored, and overly indulged. Sexual partners have become products, and the range of sexual experiences offered by modern life is limited, flattened, and holds no fascination. Women aren't experiencing orgasms as often as they should, because most of the sex they have is fleeting and detached. They engage in sex as if it's a transaction, faking an orgasm just to get it over with or not reaching climax because their partner couldn't care less. Men don't want to take the time or effort to please them. Strangers hook up in bathroom stalls or any place that's expedient. They leave unsatisfied, but it's not their bodies that are empty, it's their spirits. This has created a new kind of impotence. The hunger for even greater thrills goes unmet, pushing women to do things they're not comfortable with just because they think this is what sexual liberation looks like. Rarely is trust earned, or familiarity gained. It is much more difficult to forge a human connection, to become lost in another's eyes, to feel love as it should be felt. Just bodies against bodies. Only a moment spent, then emptiness. We've returned, in a way, to the age of the "purse."

The sexual revolution has been derailed. A woman's sexuality has been reduced once more to a functional tool, but this time it isn't used for procreation. It's merely used. The sexual revolution was subverted. It didn't set sex free. It killed it. It didn't lead to the liberation of women. It led to their degradation. Women hoped to be equal to men, and in so many ways, they are. Feminism has played a powerful role in achieving women's rights, but it went wrong when "equality" became "sameness." The message of the sexual revolution wasn't just "Sexuality is good and natural," but, "You can have sex just like a man."

RABBI SHMULEY

The problem is that men and women are not the same—especially when it comes to sex. Men are much more able to have disconnected sex. They can jump in and out of bed because they compartmentalize in a way women can't. That's in part because their sex organs are outside their body, making it easier to have sex without intimacy. Sex can be a physical act bereft of emotional investment or connection. The sexual act for them is linear—beginning and end. Get it done and disengage. For a woman, sex is an internal, inward experience. It's literally a sharing of self. Sex for them is circular and reflective. When there's disconnection, it's far less enjoyable for a woman. Emotional compartmentalization in sex is more challenging. Women are simply different, and their receptive natures seek connectivity for greater completion and wholeness.

Pamela

I believe Fromm captured it well when he wrote that we need to be skeptical when the "equality of women" is praised as a sign of progress. He wasn't opposed to women being equal with men, but he believed this quest for equality could lead to a loss of differences as we move past being equal to becoming the same.

Equality is bought at this very price: women are equal because they are not different any more. The proposition of Enlightenment philosophy, *l'ame n'a pas de sexe,* the soul has no sex, has become the general practice. The polarity of the sexes is disappearing, and with it erotic love, which is based on this polarity. Men and women become the same, not equals as opposite poles.[3]

Fromm believed our modern, mechanized age pushes for this kind of "unindividualized equality" *because it needs each person to function identically as part of the social machine, everyone obeying the commands of others while believing they're following their own desires.* "Just as modern mass production requires the standardization of commodities," *he wrote,* "so the social progress requires the standardization of man, and this standardization is called 'equality.'"[4]

This kind of equality undermines intimacy, because it's not sameness, but the differences between men and women that fuel and energize heterosexual relationships. This is not to say that everyone must conform to gender stereotypes or that there are not other ways of living in love with one another. Instead, it is to caution against throwing the baby out with the bathwater. Sexual liberation overturned inequalities between men and women that had existed for centuries, but not everything about the male–female relationship is harmful or bad. There is something ancient and powerful about the difference between the sexes that should not be discarded. It is a mistake for women to feel as if feminism requires them to renounce their femininity, or to deny themselves the opportunity to explore the possibilities of erotic love. Doing this means observing the differences between the male and the female experience.

To appreciate these differences, we need to see others for the unique individuals they are and how they're to be appreciated for their differences, not used and treated like tools for another's use. We aren't machines to be manipulated as a means to an end. We are human beings, unique in our masculinity and femininity, to be cherished and respected as we are.

Unfortunately, we live in an increasingly narcissistic culture that's training us to be heartless and desensitized, especially with the epidemic of porn addiction and selfie sex. Our culture is all about "me, me, me": Glamorized pictures are posted online to lure in "dates" or to arrange hookups in real life, where people treat each other like slabs of meat. Everyone is taking and there isn't enough giving, and often, it's the women who are degraded.

Pamela

I have seen men order women to clean floors naked, clean the pool naked, play ping-pong naked, wear mermaid outfits—just so men can get a thrill. Powerful people in the movie industry have told me to meet them in a hotel room, "and if you don't, somebody else will—and they will get the part." I have refused. I have been offered hundreds of thousands of dollars to "share a Jacuzzi," where it was strongly implied that sharing a Jacuzzi was not all that was intended. Men have offered me a condo and a Porsche to be their "number one girl." I refused, naively most upset at the thought there might be a number two. I have maintained my dignity and self-respect on my terms.

That's what women are losing in this free-for-all, and that's why we—a rabbi and *Playboy* star—want better for them. Women want sexual liberty, but many have received sexual abuse, humiliation, and neglect instead. They're also experiencing a new kind of loneliness. Despite being more connected through social media, having more opportunities, and being liberated sexually from the labels and stereotypes of a paternalistic culture, women are increasingly lonely—and so are men. According to one study, 60 percent of women feel isolated (even as they're surrounded by people), and 20 percent say they feel like this all the time.[5] Other research has found that the number of people in America—men and women—who say they have no one to talk to about important issues nearly tripled from 1985 to 2004.[6]

Loneliness has become a modern-day epidemic. John Cacioppo, author of *Loneliness: Human Nature and the Need for Social Connection*, found that more people report chronic loneliness than they did decades ago. In the 1970s, 11 percent of Americans said they felt lonely. In 2010, that number jumped to around 45 percent in an AARP study. Cacioppo's study found it to be 26 percent. That's lower, but still a significant increase. Using social media as a replacement for being with people is one of the major causes.[7]

The dehumanizing impact of the Internet coupled with a sexual revolution that lost sight of sensuality has had a devastating effect on Americans and women in particular. They're not happy in their marriages. They're not finding connection in their most intimate relationships. They're expected to have sex with men who don't desire them and haven't earned their trust. The men they're with have to take drugs to keep up. Their body images are a wreck, as is their self-esteem. They're exhausted, and they aren't satisfied with their sex lives because there's no emotional connection. They have satisfying careers, but often this diminishes time spent with their partners, so sex is pushed to the back burner.

A sexual disconnect has taken place between men and women as making love has become expedient and desensitized. The elegant dance that used to occur between the sexes is absent. Men aren't really wooing women as much anymore, and if they do, their intentions are often misunderstood. There's little courtship, nothing chivalrous. People are merely hooking up, or they've given up and prefer to turn on the computer instead of each other. As a result of the sexual revolution, women believe they don't need a man to help them feel fulfilled, to feel wanted. But this is far from the truth. A woman wants to be desired, and when she's in a marriage, her self-image and happiness are, to some degree, dependent on a man, just as a man's confidence and self-worth are dependent on a woman's respect for him. Together, they complement each other by giving and receiving erotic love. They aren't complete in the relationship without it.

This notion, however, has been rejected in recent decades as women have divorced their femininity from masculinity, declaring its independence and autonomy. As a result, husbands don't feel like they should tend to their wives' sensual needs. Women mourn the loss, whether they realize it or not. They're increasingly unhappy and lonely. To cope, many go looking outside their marriages for that spark. No longer are they looking to each other because a chasm has opened between them.

RABBI SHMULEY

This lack of sexual connection can have many negative effects in a marriage, not only on self-image, but also on a person's mental health. I witnessed this when a couple came to me for counseling because the wife suffered from obsessive-compulsive disorder. The husband felt like a victim of her mental illness, but when I observed them, I saw that the husband contributed greatly to the problem. He kept criticizing his wife and telling her how awful she was. No wonder she was becoming obsessive-compulsive to cope with the anxiety. She was engaging in repetitive action to try to achieve an elusive perfection—anything to counter the sense of permanent inadequacy he was making her experience. In the course of my counseling them back to health, the couple revealed that their sex life was all but dead, engaging in sex only about once every three months, though they could barely remember. Intimacy was gone. A caring woman was rejected and neglected.

I told her there isn't a woman on earth who faces that much neglect and criticism from her husband who doesn't compensate by finding a source of comfort. She was taken aback and said she would never think about cheating on her husband. But she confessed that there was a young stock boy at the supermarket who complimented her on her nails, and she found herself making an extra effort to go to the nail salon so she would have pretty nails for him. It was innocent. She never did anything untoward. But feeling noticed is not a luxury but a necessity. This woman resorted to the unexpected attentions of a stranger to bolster her self-image because she wasn't getting the attention she needed from her husband.

Pamela

I draw a literary example of this from the Japanese author Jun'ichiro Tanizaki, a favorite of the writer Henry Miller. In Tanizaki's novel, The Key, *an elderly husband contrives to cure his own impotence and thereby rekindle the fire in his marriage with a younger, sexually voracious wife who is not attracted to him. He arranges for the involvement of his daughter's suitor, after whom his wife lusts. The novel proceeds through a series of intrigues, whereby the wife allows her husband to act out his desires on her while she feigns unconsciousness, imagining herself with the suitor instead. Sexual jealousy eventually cures the husband of impotence, the couple makes love vigorously and proactively, after which the intensity becomes too much and the husband finally dies of a stroke.*[8]

The message of the sexual revolution is that women like this don't need their husbands' attentions to be happy. They don't need men to meet their emotional and sensual needs. Yes, women are independent, ambitious, and every bit as talented as men. But saying they don't crave their man's affections flies in the face of erotic love, of the need to be deeply known and loved by another person, physically and spiritually. Contrary to modern ideas about female autonomy, women need to be desired. They need to be lusted after, and men need to be free to lust after them in committed and consensual relationships without being made to feel like male desire is something depraved. Deep sexual longing in a loving relationship is vital to the well-being of that relationship. The passionate longings of the feminine must be met by the masculine. The sensuality men and women share is something both need for peace, wholeness, and happiness.

I love being a woman and all that entails. I never really wanted to be an actress. It wasn't something I chose, even though I'm grateful for it because it gives me a platform to bring attention to causes I believe in. But what I have always really wanted, from the time I was a little girl, was to be a wonderful wife and mother. I thought that was what it meant to be the ultimate woman, and I still do. If men aren't there to help women with pleasure, protection, stimulation, and growth, they might as well be alone—but they do need each other. It's not wrong to want the man to be the protector and provider.

I prefer to celebrate the distinctness of a woman—her femaleness—not lose it to androgyny. The more masculine a man is, the more female a woman can be. Opposition creates a safe place to be all those amazing things women are. Why are women, women and men, men? They're different, and if they were the same, would they really need each other? There is this pressure toward androgyny that has swept over us, at least in America, and it's all about being the same. Everything is ordered, regular, and measured. The need for the opposition between the sexes breaks down; men and women no longer have to behave as men and women.

Women should not feel pressured into abandoning their femininity if they don't want to. They need to resist pressure to conform and insist that feminine sexiness and sexuality are not cordoned off and made inaccessible for modern women. It's okay to be a homemaker, a mom, and a wife. It's okay to be a queen, a princess, and all these feminine archetypes. Women can be vulnerable, and men can learn again how to truly protect them. That starts with wooing them, earning their affection, and being worthy of keeping it.

We, as a society, might think we're more sophisticated, more evolved when it comes to sex and sexuality than before the sexual revolution, but are we? Are we better for the hookup culture, sexless marriages, the instant availability of pornography with the swipe of our fingers on a computer screen, and sexual language devoid of the elegance of the past? Instead of women being courted with graceful words of respect, they're being sent messages like these from the dating app Tinder[9]: "Do you wanna sit on my face?" "If we ever have to resort to cannibalism, guess which part of you I'm going to eat first,"[10] "Only 37 kms away from being bent over and taken from behind" or "Hey! I just wanted to say I find you very attractive. If I got to know you better, I would invite you over for a romantic dinner involving an expensive $5 bottle of wine and two and a half pizza pockets. Our dinner discussion would be most imminent involving the difference between jelly and jam. Afterwards we would make our way over to my polar bear carpet and begin adaptive role-playing to those twilight movies."[11] Doesn't quite have the same ring as Robert Browning's "Grow old along with me! The best is yet to be."

Our point is not to glorify the past but to ask, "Are we better now that we've had the sexual revolution? Is there room for more progress? Is it not time for a sensual revolution?" Let's be clear. Nobody wants to go back to a repressive past when women were treated as inferior and a woman's libido was barely acknowledged. But why were we ever forced to choose between female repression and female exploitation?

The 1960s were meant to be something wonderful, but the social disruption of the sexual revolution stripped sex of its spirituality and intimacy. Femininity became detached from any intimate longing for masculinity. Women became disconnected from men. Autonomy led to isolation. The sexual revolution started out being positive for women, with the goal to make their lives happier, more satisfying, and more fulfilling. But it has been sidetracked. This doesn't mean we should go back to how things were before the 1960s. There's no advocacy here for a new kind of prudishness that leads to oppression from others. People should enjoy sex and feel free with their sexuality. But this simple fact can't be denied: the sexual revolution, as it stands, has deprived us of the one thing it promised—sex! Instead of giving us good, fulfilling sex that brings us together as fully known individuals, the sexual revolution and its explosion in the age of the Internet has led us away from connected sensuality and into a pornographic wasteland of desensitization, exploitation, and loneliness.

CHAPTER 5

Is Porn for Losers?

Sometimes I get real lonely sleeping with you..

Haruki Murakami

Pamela

I know what it's like to be with men addicted to hardcore porn. It was degrading and hurtful. I thought I was the only one who experienced being neglected and played with like that—it was a kind of abuse. It was confusing—and controlling. I knew I was going to have to get out of that situation. It was difficult, though. I tried, but I couldn't fix them. I also realized maybe they were happy that way—it's a free world. It just wasn't for me. I wasn't to blame. They weren't to blame. But I needed a romantic life. I needed sensuality and kindness. I needed to be free to explore and be known. I would read Frida Kahlo, "You deserve a lover who . . . never gets tired of studying your expressions . . . who listens when you sing . . . who takes away the lies and brings you hope, coffee, and poetry,"[1] and I would think, "This definitely isn't it." I needed someone who wanted to touch a living, breathing woman, someone who wouldn't keep vanishing into the abyss of technology, someone who didn't feel like they'd been replaced by a machine, unfeeling and distant. Even though there was more to this situation than porn addiction, I believe an addiction to pornography does not help any relationship.

A lot of people, however, think hardcore porn is just for fun, that it's merely a "curiosity." Some think it helps people have better sex, but this is a mistake. Pornography—especially the online hardcore pornography of today—is a depiction of sex according to the priorities of a profit-driven industry. Pornographic sex is distorted, degraded, cheapened. Porn-informed sex is the worst kind of sex. People whose ideas about sex have been shaped by porn will not understand how to make love to another person. The sexiness of real lovemaking—connecting with another flesh-and-blood human being—is absent in porn.

Yet, porn is becoming all too pervasive in our culture. In a report by Pornhub, one of the top video pornography sites on the Internet, only one percent of its traffic came from mobile phones and tablets in 2008. That number increased to 75 percent in 2017. In 2007, when the site was first launched, 134 hours of pornographic videos had been uploaded for viewing. That exploded to 476,921 hours in 2016. Pornography is a growing multi-billion-dollar industry that's negatively affecting the lives of young and old alike, gay and straight, married and single. And it's destroying relationships.

We're not just making a wild assertion. Research and experts on sex and sexual trauma support our claim. In a 2016 study on the "Longitudinal Effects of Pornography Use On Divorce," participants who were interviewed in three "study waves" said pornography use negatively affected their marriage. "Beginning pornography use between survey waves nearly doubled one's likelihood of being divorced by the next survey period, from 6 percent to 11 percent, and nearly tripled for women, from 6 percent to 16 percent," the study's lead author reported.

The American Academy of Matrimonial Lawyers has reported that

68 percent of divorces involved one of the spouses meeting someone
new via the Internet; 56 percent involved having "an obsessive interest" in online porn; 47 percent involved spending too much time on the
computer; and 33 percent involved excessive time spent in chat rooms.[2]
Experts have testified before the U.S. Senate subcommittee on Science,
Technology, and Space about the "Brain Science Behind Pornography
Addiction and the Effects of Addiction on Families and Communities."
Judith Reisman, president of the Institute of Media Education, said that
with advances in neuroscience, we now see that porn changes how the
brain works.

> [W]e now know that emotionally arousing images imprint and alter the brain, trig-
> gering an instant, involuntary, but lasting, biochemical memory trail. Once our neu-
> rochemical pathways are established they are difficult or impossible to delete. Erotic
> images also commonly trigger the viewer's "fight or flight" sex hormones producing
> intense arousal states that appear to fuse the conscious state of libidinous arousal with
> unconscious emotions of fear, shame, anger and hostility. These media erotic fantasies
> become deeply imbedded, commonly coarsening, confusing, motivating and addict-
> ing many of those exposed. Pornography triggers a myriad of endogenous, internal,
> natural drugs that mimic the "high" from a street drug. Addiction to pornography is
> addiction to what I dub erototoxins—mind altering drugs produced by the viewer's
> own brain.[3]

As Mary Anne Layden of the Department of Psychiatry at the University of Pennsylvania testified at that same hearing:

> Pornography, by its very nature, is an equal opportunity toxin. It damages the viewer, the
> performer, and the spouses and the children of the viewers and the performers. It is toxic
> mis-education about sex and relationships. It is more toxic the more you consume, the
> "harder" the variety you consume and the younger and more vulnerable the consumer.[4]

One of these toxic effects is that it makes people less interested in their real-life partners. Both men and women who were exposed to nonviolent pornography for six weeks, with one-hour sessions each week, were less satisfied with their intimate partner's "affection, physical appearance, sexual curiosity, and sexual performance."[5] They also became more interested in "sex without emotional involvement."[6] An additional study found that porn use causes men and women to have doubts about the value of marriage and monogamy.[7]

Not only does porn devalue marriage, but it does it in the most insidious way. Even if you're happy with your relationship and enjoying sex with your partner, pornography will cause you to start thinking about alternatives.[8] The girl sitting across from you at work suddenly becomes an irresistible temptation. The stranger who stops by for a sales call at the office has taken on a new shine. You find yourself imagining him in romantic situations, even if you're already in a committed relationship. Blood rushes to your cheeks, and you start looking for ways to get him alone. Suddenly, your marriage doesn't seem as exciting. Sex with your husband or wife just isn't as satisfying as it used to be. You tell yourself it's their fault, they've allowed passion to dwindle—they're not meeting your needs. This reveals just how toxic pornography can be; it causes people to stray from or eventually become dissatisfied with perfectly good relationships.

Research confirms what many of us know from experience: watching sexually explicit materials disrupts communication between couples, makes them less dedicated to each other, and lowers sexual satisfaction.[9] People who don't watch porn at all are much happier with their relationships than those who view pornography alone *or* with their partner—so much for the myth that watching pornography together will give you that spark you need in the bedroom, an argument Rabbi Shmuley has heard so many times in counseling sessions that he can practically mouth the words along with the couple repeating it.

In one study, at least half of the participants who viewed sexually explicit materials alone *and* with their partners committed adultery.[10] Another study called "A Love That Doesn't Last: Pornography Consumption and Weakened Commitment to One's Romantic Partner" came to the same conclusion—porn weakens relationship bonds. This team found that watching porn lowered commitment to the relationship in both men and women, but it had a stronger impact on men. When the pornography was removed, commitment increased.[11] All it took was turning off the computer and spending time with their real-life partner.

When people erase the fantasies and images that stand between them, they see one another more clearly. They see the person they fell in love with. They rediscover desire for each other. No strangers, no temptations at the office, no ruminations about the inadequacies and failures of the institution of marriage, no questions about commitment to monogamy. They're free of the chains that have kept them from enjoying what they already have.

When it comes to porn, women have to be particularly aware of the effect it has on men. While studies have found that both men and women are more open to straying after viewing porn, this impacts men a lot more than women, as does relationship dissatisfaction in general. While many women can watch porn and still maintain intimacy with their partner, men struggle to do the same. Their thoughts are fixated on images more than women's are. One study found that men considered their partners less attractive after viewing sexually explicit pictures of other women.[12]

Researchers believe this is because exposure to these images causes men to undergo a kind of rewiring in their brain about what a typical naked body should look like.[13] So while women might be able to view porn and honestly say it doesn't affect how they view their partner, they can't assume the same is true for their guy. He might not admit it or even realize it, but studies have shown this to be true and it fits with a man's highly visual nature. If a woman doesn't want another woman in her partner's thoughts, she shouldn't tolerate him watching porn—not when he's alone or even with her.

Porn not only affects relationship quality, but it can also decrease sexual function. According to Layden, men who watch a lot of pornography tend to have problems with premature ejaculation and erectile dysfunction. Having spent so much time in unnatural sexual experiences with celluloid and cyberspace, they seem to find it difficult to have sex with a real human being. Pornography is raising their expectation and demand for types and amounts of sexual experiences at the same time it is reducing their ability to experience sex.[14]

A 2016 study found that erectile dysfunction, delayed ejaculation, and diminished libido during sex in men under forty can be caused by pornography.[15] The study looked at how the brain's motivational system is altered by viewing porn and postulated that Internet pornography, with its "limitless novelty, potential for easy escalation to more extreme material, video format, etc.," could be powerful enough to condition sexual arousal in such a way that sex with real-life partners doesn't live up to expectations.[16] And the more sexual images men and women absorb, the more they move from "subjective attraction," colored by love and the emotions, to "objective attraction," determined by an expertise in the human body that is rarely healthy to acquire. How many women begin to feel that their bodies are inadequate not intrinsically but in comparison to others? Too many.

Consider how these changes in expectations manifest in marriages. The relationship starts to collapse before either of the spouses realizes what's happening or why. A woman begins to notice her husband is more critical of her looks, her weight, how she dresses. Or, if he doesn't say anything negative, he doesn't compliment either. Her new hairstyle goes unnoticed. The dress she bought just for him is worn without a second glance. During sex—when they have it—he's disconnected and insensitive. He's less concerned about getting her needs met. Gradually, he begins to suggest they do new and "fun" things in the bedroom. Not because he wants to have greater passion with her, but because he's acting out a deperson-alized fantasy. She's a little hesitant, but she does it—just to please him. He seems to like it for a while, but then he gets bored. He then either pulls away or decides to do something else that's even more "creative," but this time she's not comfortable with it. She tries, but he knows she's not into it. Eventually, they stop having sex. One, two, six months go by, and he hasn't touched her. She gets word through a mutual friend that he blames *her* for the lack of sex. She internalizes the guilt and maybe even believes it.

This scenario is repeated all too often, and the root of it is exposure to porn of some form or another. A hopeful finding, which is confirmed in several studies, is that when people stop watching Internet porn, these negative effects can often be reversed.[17] There can be real love and desire once more. But it takes rewiring the brain and forming new habits.

One concern about the effect of porn on the brain is that our children are exposed to pornography at increasingly younger ages. Pornography has always been around, but there was a time when people didn't view sexu-ally explicit materials until they were older. The most a child or a teenager would see was a glimpse of a centerfold kept under their uncle's bed or the grainy images of porn on the television screen late at night. Now, kids see crystal clear images of sexually explicit porn for the first time around the average age of twelve, with 93 percent of boys and 62 percent of girls being exposed to porn before the age of eighteen.[18] And it's not just "porn with a story" or erotica they're watching; they're potentially deluged with orgies, glory holes, hardcore porn, sadism and masochism, gang rapes, bestiality, and any other fetish you can imagine. Boys especially are being caught in the porn trap, with twelve- and seventeen-year-old males view-ing porn more frequently than anyone else.[19]

The impact of this on how young people view sex and sexual relation-ships is devastating. It's exposing them to violent sex and abuse of women. It's normalizing insensitive, aberrant sex, which makes it more likely that they will engage in similar degrading behaviors[20] or at least be dissatisfied with sex that doesn't meet expectations later in life. It's affecting their self-image, as they compare their bodies to those they see on the screen—this is especially damaging to girls who suffer from body image issues. It's influencing them to use coarse and demeaning language, particularly toward women. It's also introducing them to a need to push boundaries even in the earliest stages of sexual exploration, as with anal sex, which has increased among teenagers in recent years. A small study of British heterosexual teenagers in 2014 discovered some disturbing trends on this point. It found that while most teens were having anal sex within a relationship, some first experiences rarely involved cooperative exploration:[21]

Instead, it was mainly men who pushed the women to try anal sex, and men said they felt expected to take this role. Moreover, the teens expected men to find pleasure in anal sex, whereas women were mostly expected to endure the negative aspects of anal sex, such as pain or a damaged reputation.[22]

While young women in the study complained about anal sex being painful, most teenagers said that's because women are "naive or flawed" and "unable to relax."[23] Young men in the study admitted they were inspired to try anal sex because they wanted to mimic what they saw in pornography, and they "appeared to perceive having anal sex as a feat in competition."[24] The challenge was to persuade or coerce girls into doing it. The young women confirmed this when they admitted seeing "their role as accepting or declining their partner's request for anal sex, rather than being an equal decision-maker about this sexual activity."[25]

Another effect of porn is a decline in sexual activity among late Millennials and iGens. Compared to earlier generations, including Millennials born in the 1980s and early 1990s, young people are having sex less, and one of the reasons is pornography and lack of face-to-face interaction due to use of computers and smartphones. According to a recent study,

15 percent of twenty- to twenty-four-year-olds haven't had sex as adults compared to 6 percent in the 1990s.[26] Significantly, this is the generation raised on smartphones from an early age. Norman Spack, an associate professor at Harvard Medical School, said the way young people communicate today is "anti-sexual"—"People are not spending enough time alone just together," he said. "There's another gorilla in the room: It's whatever is turned on electronically."[27] Comments by an eighteen-year-old interviewed by *The Washington Post* supports Spack's explanation:

> Noah Patterson, 18, likes to sit in front of several screens simultaneously: a work project, a YouTube clip, a video game. To shut it all down for a date or even a one-night stand seems like a waste. "For an average date, you're going to spend at least two hours, and in that two hours I won't be doing something I enjoy," he said. It's not that he doesn't like women. "I enjoy their companionship, but it's not a significant part of life," said Patterson, a Web designer in Bellingham, Wash. He has never had sex, although he likes porn. "I'd rather be watching YouTube videos and making money." Sex, he said, is "not going to be something people ask you for on your résumé."[28]

Kids having less sex is a good thing, but we have to look at the reason why, and for this youngest generation, at least one of the reasons is a lack of connection with other people due to technology and the use of pornography. That's not the best motivation people should have to refrain from sex—or even dating.

Pamela

I was keenly aware of these trends when I was bringing up my two boys. Concerned that they were growing up in a world without romance, I raised them as romantics. I taught them romance isn't just about the woman you're with; it's about having a romantic life, being engaged with the world. It's about having empathy, loving nature and art, and caring about things outside yourself. Having taught my boys these values, I now have complete faith in their ability to treat their relationships properly.

Learning is a two-way street, of course, even between parents and children. I learned from my boys, too. Once, when I was teaching my son Brandon about the importance of respect, I told him, "If you don't respect women, you don't respect me." *He answered,* "But what if they don't respect themselves?" *That was an interesting point, and I agreed that women have to respect and love themselves always.*

Genuine, healthy relationships are impossible if that doesn't happen, not just for women, but men as well. Watching Internet porn videos isn't respecting yourself or others. It desensitizes instead of enlivens. It robs relationships of intimacy and passion, deadening the relationship. Pornography needs to be taken seriously because it's robbing people of the joy of sensual sex. Kids are growing up thinking sex is disconnected, painful, demeaning to women, involving many partners,[29] and even violent. Porn is making them less interested in connecting with real people. This doesn't mean every person who has ever watched pornography will be dissatisfied with their relationships, but the trends aren't looking good. We want children to be free of the damaging and degrading effects of porn, so they don't carry baggage into their future relationships. We want men and women to be free to express themselves in a sensual and connected way, one that will enrich and strengthen their marriages. We want them to rediscover the sexual tension they once had in their relationship and remember the thrill of making love.

CHAPTER 6

Loosening Sexual Tension

Poetry is a naked woman, a naked man, and the distance between them.

LAWRENCE FERLINGHETTI

J oseph Campbell once wrote, "Hell is life drying up." The same can be said of marriage. It's hell when there's no life in it. Integral to life is energy, animation, and tension. For a marriage to be alive, there needs to be sexual tension. There needs to be *oomph*. Marriages are dying because the bonds of sexual tension have been loosened, relaxed to the point of nonexistence. Desire has shriveled, and it has been replaced with the tranquility of companionship and friendship. There's nothing wrong with friendship in marriage, but if there's no passion, then there's no intensity. When this happens, husbands and wives turn outward to feel that sexual tension—habitual flirtation, pornography, and affairs. Or they just give up and go numb, living together with cool detachment.

Sadly, some think it's supposed to be this way. They might even take pride in it. They put all their energy into work, caring for the home, or raising children, thinking this is the essence of marriage. Others look to religion as justification for killing desire. They hold to a practical dualism that pits the spirit against the flesh, rejecting the idea that passion is necessary in marriage—it's all about duty. Erotic love, for them, has been reduced to an obligation, a responsibility.

This only adds to the false notion that marriage is a graveyard of desire. Not willing to live as zombies, some people are abandoning monogamy altogether, replacing it with unhealthy and inevitably destructive arrangements such as open marriages or multipartner relationships known as polyamory. These people think they're offering a viable solution to the problem of broken marriages. Instead of cheating and breaking up, they say, you should just admit that the monogamy thing isn't working, accept the truth, stay together, but look to other people to fill in the gaps, to be the spark that reignites the marriage. Anything else, they say, runs counter to human nature.

While it's certainly true that human beings naturally find it difficult to be monogamous, we don't simply act on instinct or emotions. We are rational creatures, and we can *choose* to love and desire only one person if we set our minds to it. It just takes effort, but that effort doesn't mean merely digging in and enduring a lifeless marriage for the sake of staying together. It means working to reignite passion and maintaining it within the marriage.

Believe it or not, you can have a relationship electrified by sexual tension if you want it. You can be married to one person and keep the burning fires of lust alive. You don't have to have an open marriage or litter your home with several partners. And you don't have to endure a sexless marriage where you feel dead inside. Plenty of couples have done it—they've kept the flames of romantic desire lit.

Pamela

My parents are a prime example. They've been through tough times; they're friends, companions, caretakers, but they've never stopped desiring each other.

They're playful, full of life, and passionate. They're committed soul mates. Their love has never died because their lust for each other has been kept alive. That's the example set for me, that's my ideal, and that's what I want for myself, my children, and everyone else.

RABBI SHMULEY

That's what I want for the many couples I meet who are despondent and hopeless that their marriages can change. I want them to breathe new life into their relationships. I've seen it happen many times—a marriage teetering on the edge of a cliff brought back to sure footing through commitment, hard work, and a willingness to embrace sexual tension. Sometimes eroticism is lost because of work, other interests, distractions, or, more often than not, the arrival of children.

This happened to one couple I counseled, whose marriage started out full of romance, but then they had babies. After that, the game was over. No more intimacy. No more passion. The wife wanted the children with them all the time, even in bed at night. She nursed them long after most women stop. Eventually, the husband moved to the couch, and over time, he lost interest in his wife. Instead of being erotic, her body became functional. He admired her as a mother; in fact he thought she was the greatest mother in the world. But as a wife and sexual partner—that had almost ceased to exist.

I didn't want to judge the wife on her parenting choices, but I did tell her that if the children were always in the bed, she and her husband would have no romantic getaway—and they needed it. She began to realize this and make a change, but a child in the bedroom wasn't the only issue in the marriage. The husband had embraced complacency. He didn't like that he and his wife were no longer intimate and passionate, but he had stopped putting forth the effort to make it happen. He just moved to the couch and gave up. He had allowed himself to stop seeing his wife erotically. It was easier, in a way, to see her only as a maternal figure. He missed having sex, but he wasn't willing to expend the energy to work at it. He wasn't willing to embrace the sexual tension that comes with maintaining eroticism in a marriage.

Think of all the work a man puts into a relationship while dating. He is constantly full of anxiety about the woman he wants. He worries about anyone else she's with, works hard to get her attention, and exhausts himself trying to win her over. That shouldn't stop when they get married or even after children are born. This needs to be maintained in marriage, but it takes energy. It takes commitment. This man had failed to do that. To fix the relationship, he needed to do the hard work of embracing sexual tension and the danger that comes with eroticism.

I explained that one way he could do that was to ask his wife if she had sexual needs. She worked half days and was gone from home—did she ever have sexual fantasies? Had any other man ever looked at her as a woman, a sexual creature? The purpose of asking this, I told him, was to begin to see his wife once again not just as a wife but as a woman. Not just as a mother but as a sexual being. Seeing her through the eyes of other men could help with this.

The wife admitted that there were two men in her office who would talk to her and send her funny emails. One was always telling her humorous stories, making her laugh. She liked how he made her feel. The husband started to get angry because she hadn't told him this before. She quipped back, *"Because you'd get angry, just like you are now!"* He didn't like the anxiety it caused to be married to an erotic woman. It was easier just to see her as a mom.

"You want a woman you can control, and you're blaming the

children for the decline in your libido," I told him. "Don't feel bad. This often happens with men, and they don't even realize it. But instead of giving over to the complacency, embrace the danger. Ask her if she ever has fantasies about other men."

"*But that's inappropriate!*" the husband said.

"Being half married is inappropriate," I responded. "Infidelity is inappropriate, but that's not what this is."

During their next session, the husband said he did as I advised. His wife told him her fantasies, but it made him uncomfortable. He stayed in the bed with her (the kids were now gone to their own rooms), but he ignored her. He admitted, however, that hearing about her fantasies did begin to change how he looked at her. He began to see her as a sexual woman again and not just as a mom to their kids. The next night, he asked her again. He was jealous, but he made love to her, and over time their sexual relationship improved. They continued along that path and embraced some of the danger that's part of being human. As their sex life improved, so did their relationship.

It seems rather simple, but why are so many couples, like this one, willing to give up and endure marriages empty of desire? It's because they're not comfortable with tension. From the time we're children, we're told to keep calm. We're protected from anything that might cause us, or our parents, to be anxious. Freedom is sacrificed in childhood for safety and harmony. Parents helicopter around their children to make sure they don't scrape their knees or get into arguments with other kids. They're not allowed to run and explore, to fall and get up again. Children never learn how to cope with stress and worry that come with being free. Boys are especially affected. They're pumped with medications because they're too full of energy and "hyperactive." The adventurousness and vitality of a child are seen as problems to be cured rather than natural tendencies to be nurtured. As they get older, many can't cope with the anxieties of life, so they're given antidepressants to dull their senses, to calm them. The side effects of many of these drugs are well known—lack of feeling, loss of libido, and at times, sexual dysfunction. How are people who are dulled by drugs supposed to maintain intense passion and feeling in their relationships?

Drugs, of course, are only part of the problem. As we've seen, our sensuality is deadened by overuse of technology, the desensitizing effects of pornography, and the hypersexualization of our culture, which diminishes sexual anticipation and removes the mystery of sex. Our modern philosophy of life, which came about through the sexual revolution, also plays a part. Men and women are treated as if they're the same—the distinctions between masculine and feminine have been blurred and, in some cases, erased. But, at least in heterosexual relationships, it's within the interplay of the masculine and feminine that sexual tension is created. If relationships blend into an androgynous unit instead of remaining two separate and very different entities, there will be a loss of friction, sexual tension, and vitality.

While compatibility is a good thing, it's not what gives relationships the energy to stay alive. Desire is the lifeblood of marriages—the deep knowing of Eros. Unfortunately, the need for tranquility, the loss of masculine and feminine distinctiveness, and an overvalued sense of friendship in marriage has killed sexual tension. The result is a marital wasteland where wives feel depleted and depressed and men endure a monotonous existence that's draining their energy and zest for life. Husbands and wives rush through the busyness of the day, keeping themselves occupied with the necessities of life so they don't have to feel the despair that's seeping into their spirits. When they do step away from work, they flood their minds with family duties or entertainment and sports. In the blue glow of a screen, life loses it kaleidoscopic vitality. At the end of the day, they fall into bed, wondering where the day went and why they aren't happier.

They look at their spouse and feel little desire. They feel love. They might even talk for a while and hold each other, but the passion is gone. If they have sex, it's listless and routine.

Why can't they make the passion last from one year to the next? Is there hope that in their old age they will be together, still in love with romance in their eyes? Or will they be lonely like so many are today? Is this the destiny of marriage? Is it the institution that's the problem? Or did they simply marry the wrong person? Or is the very notion of love a myth?

Pamela

I've spoken to men who have asked these questions, having become disillusioned with marriage. "The sex was boring; there was no spark," they tell me. "It was a chore." So they divorced, swearing never to marry again. They hang out with their friends and get their sexual needs met by prostitutes, someone new every day or week; those who remain married lie to their wives. There's no intimacy and no connection. They think this is the best they can do.

RABBI SHMULEY

As a child of divorce, I've spent my life trying to get men and women to believe and invest in their marriages again, so kids don't end up in the situation I found myself in at the tender age of eight. But I have no desire to keep people in the cold prison of a loveless marriage. Rather, I want to make marriage passionate and intimate and even "naughty" again.

How many people have you seen living in a dead marriage where they're beaten down, resigned to a life of dreariness? If you ask them what's wrong, they'll say they just feel worn out. They try to figure out why, but they don't really know. So many people are tired, but it's not because they're busy working two jobs to make ends meet. This might cause some physical fatigue, but it doesn't explain the sad loneliness and despair that is becoming an epidemic in our time. What people are feeling is spiritual fatigue, a weariness in their souls because they have little vitality. They're caught in a vicious cycle of keeping anxiety and despair at bay by being busy, but the rat race of a material world generates even more despair. By shutting down the spirit and focusing only on physical needs and responsibilities, or smothering it with passive entertainment, people are not truly living. They have no freedom of spirit. They aren't invigorated by dreams, expectations, and the rush of life. They are caught in a trap.

People need to be free, to live again, to feel a new lust for life and for each other. Couples need to experience the thrill of eroticism, of the sexual tension and the vibrancy of being alive. But these couples can't if they're suffering from spiritual impotence. They can't know the passion that overflows into every crack and crevice of life. They can't feel the sensual delights of the person they love because there is no fire. They want to feel it, but they look backward instead of forward. They long for the days when they were seventeen, the sun on their faces, the wind in their hair, the scent of autumn, and the hope of new love with a new school year, their imaginations burning to explore and know. They remember falling in love with the object of their desire—those first kisses, the hesitancy, the longing. The sexual tension between them was palpable. They could taste it, smell it, feel it, breathe it in. There was electricity between them because they were alive.

Do you want to feel alive again, to feel the intensity of human connection, the electricity of human touch? Are you weary of a meaningless existence in which you're not living, but only surviving—one day after another, a boring slog instead of an exciting adventure? Do you want desire to course through your veins once more? It can. You can feel that way again—your marriage doesn't have to be lifeless. Where there is love, there is hope, but simply coexisting, carrying out the mundane demands of daily life, and sharing a benign friendship won't make it happen. You need to look beyond the routine physical and dive into the depths of the soul. You need to rediscover desire and unlock the mysteries of the erotic mind.

Part Two

WHAT HAPPENED TO
EROTIC LOVE?

CHAPTER 7

Too Much of a Good Thing

Take a lover that looks at you like maybe you are magic.

FRIDA KAHLO

S he took her bra off as casually as if she were undressing to go to sleep," a young college student told Rabbi Shmuley. "It was like she had done it a million times. It was so easy. No mystery, no hesitancy, no trembling anticipation, no nervous excitement. There was nothing coy about it. Just stripping down, having sex, then it was done. I sat there stunned by how nonchalant it was. It left me numb."

He said it wasn't what he imagined it would be. Sex was so common; it had lost its allure and the rush that comes with doing something forbidden. It was like eating a meal; each hookup is just one more bite on the plate. You hardly finish tasting the first before moving on to the second. You never even feel hunger pangs because you're filling and refilling so quickly. There's nothing special about it, because there's no emotional connection with the person who should make it special. There's just sex, and more sex.

While this isn't the experience of everyone, it's far too common today.

Our society is saturated in sex—a complete turnaround since the 1950s when sex was hidden in the shadows and inhibition defined eroticism even in marriage. The sexual revolution was a logical rebellion against that warped perception of sex. The shadows created shame and dysfunction. That was the problem. The solution offered by the sexual revolution was to bring sex into the open. The more we exposed our sexuality, the more we experimented, the more uninhibited we became, the better sex we'd have—and the happier we would be. That was the promise.

So we threw open the floodgates of unrestrained sex—counterculture movements, sexually liberal attitudes, relaxation of censorship laws, free love, and the Golden Age of Porn all came rushing into the mainstream. Andy Warhol's *Blue Movie*, Bill Osco's *Mona* played by Fifi Watson, and Gerard Damiano's *Deep Throat* starring Linda Lovelace blazed the trail for erotic film. Pornography burst from the shadows. Meanwhile, sexual liberation, energized by second-wave feminism, ripped through the artistic community and into the American psyche.

Even when the Supreme Court redefined obscenity in 1973 and held that the First Amendment does not protect it[1]—a decision that made it easier for states to prosecute sellers of obscene material—the porn industry survived. With the court's ruling, erotic film was driven from the big screen to small, low-budget venues, but this didn't reduce public consumption of porn. It merely changed the vehicle of distribution, and with the widespread use of videocassettes in the 1980s and the Internet a decade later, its availability and acceptability hit a saturation point, allowing people to consume pornography in the privacy of their own homes.

The sexual revolution sought to normalize sexuality and enrich relationships, but over time and with advances in technology generating greater access, it has been subverted, leading to the deterioration of sexuality and the weakening of relationships. Sex has been reduced to a mere physical transaction that's readily available with the stroke of a computer key. The fire of desire has diminished, the magic of sensuality has increasingly disappeared, the wonder of sexual exploration and curiosity has faded, leaving us detached and desensitized. Sex is supposed to be an intimate, romantic, fun experience, not just a mechanical release. It's supposed to make us feel alive. But overexposure ruins sex, robbing it of vitality. Sex is meant to be intense and primal, an explosion of color, a vibrant moment captured and shared. But when you remove mystery, anticipation, longing, and sensuality, good sex withers and dies.

Nothing reveals this better than a 2015 *Vanity Fair* article, "Tinder and the Dawn of the 'Dating Apocalypse'" by Nancy Jo Sales, in which she interviews several men and women in a Manhattan bar who use dating apps like Tinder.[2] With just a swipe of the finger, they go through dozens of potential hookups in just an hour. "[Y]ou're always sort of prowling," one man said. "You could talk to two or three girls at a bar and pick the best one, or you can swipe a couple hundred people a day—the sample size is so much larger. It's setting up two or three Tinder dates a week and, chances are, sleeping with all of them, so you could rack up 100 girls you've slept with in a year."[3]

"Dating apps are the free-market economy come to sex," Sales writes.[4] It's all about instant gratification. "Sex has become so easy," one man said. "I can go on my phone right now and no doubt I can find someone I can have sex with this evening, probably before midnight."[5]

Hookups like these have left some people feeling devalued and disrespected. The one thing Sales heard from the men she interviewed was, "Too easy," "Too easy," "Too easy."[6] There's no respect, and there's scant erotic desire because you can't pine for something that's already in the palm of your hand. Men aren't the only ones to blame. Women put themselves in the position to be treated disrespectfully because they think it's the best they can do or they just want to go along with the crowd. Apps like Tinder are extensions of more general social media like Facebook, which encourage people to turn themselves into products, to sell themselves like trinkets at a fire sale. Each person is unique and unquantifiable, but the dating economy dangles sex in front of people's noses, and then forces them to conform, to list their assets and put themselves on a market, in order to get that sex. Everything is focused on the next fix, the next sale, not the development of enduring human bonds. The result is a sex-frenzied melee that does nothing to promote healthy relationships or develop good lovers.

Christopher Ryan, co-author of *Sex at Dawn*, told Sales that what's happening in the online dating scene mirrors the pattern we've seen with porn:[7] "The appetite has always been there, but it had restricted availability; with new technologies the restrictions are being stripped away and we see people sort of going crazy with it. I think the same thing is happening with this unlimited access to sex partners. People are gorging. That's why it's not intimate. You could call it a kind of psychosexual obesity."[8]

RABBI SHMULEY

One young woman I counseled found herself caught in this web of nonintimate sex and the suffering that goes with it. She grew up in a traditional home, but she met a man unlike any she had ever known. He was deeply emotional and played on her feelings. In truth, he was a seduction artist and had a girlfriend. She was just one more notch in his belt, but she fell for him. She gave him her virginity. Not long after, he became abusive and then cut her off, refusing to answer her phone calls. Desperate to discover what was wrong, she went over to his house. He started yelling at her and demeaning her. He was done with her. He used her then discarded her like yesterday's newspaper. The girl fell into deep depression. The whole memory of it became loathsome to her. She felt like a fool. Her first sexual experience was a meaningless, nonintimate connection, and loss of innocence like this inevitably breeds contempt. She soon began talking about how much she distrusted men.

Examples like this show an immature form of love, which Erich Fromm called "symbiotic union."[9] This is a form of love, he says, where one person becomes masochistic and the other person becomes sadistic. The sadist "wants to escape from his aloneness and his sense of imprisonment by making another person part and parcel of himself." He "commands, exploits, hurts, humiliates."[10] On the other hand, the masochist tries to "escape from the unbearable feeling of isolation and separateness by making [her]self part and parcel of another person."[11] She has no self-worth except when she is exploited, and in doing so comes to be dominated by the sadist. Both people are harmed by this kind of relationship, but it is increasingly common in today's society.

Promiscuity often causes pain and bitterness because it keeps people from forming relationships organically. For that to happen, you need to go through four stages of development: attraction, verbal exploration, emotional intimacy, and physical intimacy. When you put physical intimacy first or second, you never really get to know the person, and you never experience emotional intimacy. You've just become one more person to be devoured in a culture that glorifies sex for the sake of sex.

Oversexualization breeds dysfunction. In the American culture, this starts at a young age, as sexualizing and pornographic messaging, particularly from the Internet and movies, push children to become sexually active before they're "emotionally, socially or intellectually ready."[12] Years before they even hit their eighteenth birthday, their perceptions about sex become informed, not by parental instruction or personal experience in a committed relationship, but by consumer-driven, artificial sexual messaging.

Pornography is especially destructive since the average age for first-time exposure is twelve and these early impressions about sex do not change over time. Jean Twenge, an expert on sexual trends in America, notes "that adolescents and young adults form their views around sexuality at earlier stages of development and do not alter them much beyond their formative development years."[13] Early exposure to pornography is like feeding children plastic food and expecting them to grow up healthy. It won't happen.

Oversexualization has long-term negative effects, particularly on those who have sex early. Studies have shown that "children who have sex by the age of 13 are more likely to have multiple sexual partners, engage in frequent intercourse, have unprotected sex and use drugs or alcohol before sex."[14] Other research shows that "more than 66 percent of boys and 40 percent of girls reported wanting to try some of the sexual behaviors they saw in the media (and by high school, many had done so)."[15]

A report from the American Psychological Association Task Force on the Sexualization of Girls found that overexposure of sex hits women especially hard.[16] They're more prone to body image issues, depression, and low self-esteem. If sexualization leads to self-objectification, their cognitive ability is decreased and they experience feelings of shame. "This cognitive diminishment, as well as the belief that physical appearance rather than academic or extracurricular achievement is the best path to power and acceptance, may influence girls' achievement levels and opportunities later in life."[17]

A girl's sexual development is also negatively affected, as her self-perception about virginity and having sex for the first time is influenced by a sexualizing media. Her relationship with other girls is often disrupted. They either support or turn on each other depending on how much they conform to a narrow ideal about sexualized beauty or who can get the attention of boys. And when it comes to boys, their views on dating become sexualized, and boys feel freer to sexually harass women or even become violent.[18]

Oversexualization narrows what men find attractive in a woman, making "it difficult for some men to find an 'acceptable' partner or to fully enjoy intimacy with a female partner."[19] In particular, exposure to pornography "leads men to rate their female partners as less attractive, to indicate less satisfaction with their intimate partners' attractiveness, sexual performance, and level of affections, and to express greater desire for sex without emotional involvement."[20]

And that's not the only problem. Younger men who typically don't experience erectile dysfunction are turning to drugs to overcome desensitization due to watching too much porn. Drugs also help them get past psychological insecurities and inhibitions they face when meeting women who are driven to have sex more than they ever have been.[21] Men don't want to be judged when compared to the images women see on a screen (in the same way women don't).

"There is an increased anxiety among young men because this generation of women is more open to erotica, more articulate about their own needs," a clinical psychologist and sex therapist at Beth Israel Medical Center told *The New York Times*.[22] "That contributes to men's anxiety, because they think they're being evaluated in a different way."[23] She said young men are using drugs as "psychological safety nets" because they have bought into the myth that "the man is always interested in sex, always ready to go and having to be a quote-unquote superman."[24] And if they want to have kinky sex or do anything they're not used to, the drugs can provide the fuel to keep it going.[25] It's not about being driven by passion for your partner. It's not about desire for another human being. It's about the act—a medically induced performance masquerading as great sex.

This is true not only for straight men, but for gay men as well. Many gay men are made to feel as if they need to go on for hours and hours because that's what the "adventure" of sex is all about—or so they believe. Just like with the heterosexual population, that's what one porno after another has told them. That's the goal. And if they want to live up to porn-defined expectations, then they turn to drugs to alleviate their fears of failure.[26]

What's lost in all this is an actual relationship with another person. Medications can be more of a hindrance than a help in that area. This was the case with a forty-three-year-old man who took Viagra and spent a "sex-crazed week" with a model at a hotel. The relationship didn't survive more than a few days after the trip.[27] "She had no idea what made me superman," the man said in an interview with *The New York Times*. "It was just unfortunate that we didn't have much to talk about afterwards."[28]

Pamela

I feel that the LGBT community may be leading the way out of this sexual alienation of modern life. A conversation I had in Paris with a gay man, a ballet dancer, bears this out. "I feel like gay people are having their sexual revolution now," he said. He explained that for so long it had been hard to find someone who wanted to be faithful in a relationship, and he felt like he was going to end up alone. There were too many stereotypes—harmful stereotypes, he felt—about the ephemeral, promiscuous nature of gay sexuality. As a gay man, he had even taken those stereotypes seriously but had never been happy. What he wanted—what everyone wants—was a loving romantic relationship of mutual support and passion. He saw the series of victories on marriage reform for the LGBT community as a positive change, because it was addressing those stereotypes, showing the world that gay people want the same things straight people do, and making it easier for gay men to find happiness.

People want to find someone to grow old with. To appreciate this, I encourage people to watch one of my favorite movies, Amour, about an elderly couple who love each other and make compassionate end-of-life decisions for each other. Many men, including gay men, have also shared with me their fears of never having a relationship. They're tired of one sex partner after another, and they're afraid they'll end up alone. Who will grow old with them? Who will care for them when they're sick? Who will walk with them through the adventure of life as they pass through the changes of every stage?

This is their worry, and yet our culture is failing them. Over the past forty years, sex in America has exploded, but it hasn't led to healthy relationships, intense sensuality, or good sex—just more bad sex or, in some cases, no sex at all. Americans in general are having more casual sex than ever: "Among 18- to 29-year-olds reporting non-partner sex, 35% of GenX'ers in the late 1980s had sex with a casual date or pickup (44% of men, 19% of women), compared to 45% of Millennials in the 2010s (55% of men, 31% of women)."[29] The number of partners has also increased. In the late 1980s, people over the age of eighteen had 7.17 sexual partners (11.42 for men, 3.54 for women), compared to 11.22 partners after 2010 (18.22 for men, 5.55 for women).[30]

The only deviation from this is a decline in sexual partners among Millennials/iGens compared to those born in the 1950s and 1960s. But even these young people still have "more sexual partners than those born in the first half of the twentieth century."[31] While some people believe there really isn't a hookup culture and that late Millennials might be ushering a new kind of sexual counterrevolution, this is not actually happening.[32] It's true that people born after the mid 1990s (late Millennials and iGens) aren't having as much sex as Boomers and early GenXers,[33] but this isn't due to a resurgence of traditional mores or a revival of healthy sexuality. It's due to a variety of factors including individualization and detachment from community, social anxieties caused by parental overprotection, and depersonalization created by overuse of technology.[34] Many people simply don't have sex because it's easier to release sexual energies with technology than with another person.

Those who do have sex aren't happy either because the sex they're having is unsatisfying. A sociology researcher at Occidental College, who has studied the college hookup scene, says casual sex is unfulfilling because it hasn't met students' "most basic desires."[35] Her research found that "the three things students were looking for in hookups were pleasure, connection, and empowerment," she said during a seminar on "Hooking Up on

Campus." "Just one of those would have been enough."[36] But hooking up doesn't meet any of these desires. Students aren't getting the emotional connection they want. Many of them don't even realize there's a problem because they're told by the hookup culture that they "must enjoy casual sex and have an active disinterest in your partner."[37] Yet, this isn't what they really need. They need their human desires met by connecting with another person, but overexposure of sex has made that difficult, leaving them dispirited and disappointed without really understanding why.

RABBI SHMULEY

Many people don't realize something is wrong until they hear a message that flies in the face of the one being sold by the culture. This happened to a man who came to one of my lectures on passionate connection. After it was over, the man asked me if we could talk. Even though the man wasn't a womanizer by nature, he said he kept finding himself in situations where he was just sleeping with one woman after another. His friends were doing it, so he did too. It wasn't anything to brag about. It just happened. But he felt like he was losing himself. *"If I go to bed with one more stranger,"* he said, *"I'll no longer know who I am. Every time I sleep with someone, I feel like I lose a piece of myself. I forget who I really am."*

Sex is knowledge. When two people have sex, there isn't any filter between them. Sex becomes a mirror. Both people come to a deeper understanding of themselves. But if sex is between strangers, it leads to invisibility. You don't see anything reflected, and you start becoming a stranger to yourself. When you begin to lose your own self, despair seeps in. Sometimes people realize what's happening, as this young man did, but many don't. They just continue the same cycle of desensitization and depersonalization, gradually becoming invisible to themselves.

This is what is so destructive about depersonalized sex. There's no connection and no knowledge of one another. This is a growing problem among heterosexual Millennials and iGens because, reports say, they're choosing to have anal and oral sex instead of vaginal sex. As with any kind of sexual experience, in a relationship of mutual respect and commitment where a sexual and emotional connection is established, anal and oral sex can be as much a function of intimacy and connection as other forms of sexual expression. But anal and oral sex, where they occur without a relationship of mutual respect, can tend to be about the satisfaction of male desire without concern for the sexual needs of the woman. While anal sex may be pleasing for the man, on its own it is not always anatomically stimulating for the woman. And whereas both men and women can receive oral sex, a greater burden of expectation usually lies on the woman to give oral sex to the man, and as a result, in heterosexual couples, it is often a one-way street.

Where sex is more about the satiation of the man's needs, this can lead to a loss of intimacy and depersonalization. Furthermore, anal and oral sex have a particular connotation in online hardcore pornography, where to receive oral sex is understood as empowering for a man and to give it is demeaning for a woman. The same is true with anal sex, which is often presented in porn as a praiseworthy desecration of a woman by a man. There is a misogynistic emphasis to the way oral and anal sex are presented in online heterosexual pornography, and when young people copy what they see in porn, they run the risk of reproducing this harmful emphasis, which only adds to the depersonalization.

So while Millennials and iGens report having less "sex" than Boomers and GenXers,[38] they're most likely having as many sexual encounters; the difference is they're not having sexual intercourse as often as older generations did. They're also probably not reporting anal and oral sex as "sex," while the Boomers and GenXers would call it sex and check the yes box on a survey even if they've only had oral or anal sex.[39]

To get a picture of the extent of this new trend, one study has found that "while 81% of college students reported engaging in some sexual behavior in the context of hooking up, only 34% reported sexual intercourse during a hookup."[40] Another study found that only about a quarter of women during their first semester of college had hookups that involved vaginal sex.[41]

Journalist Peggy Orenstein has been chronicling the lives of fifteen- to twenty-year-old girls for the past two decades and has also observed this trend toward nonintimate sex. Girls, she said in an interview on National Public Radio, think they should ignore their own desires and please only their partners, removing themselves from the experience. When it came to oral sex, they said it was something they started doing at a young age, and it was rarely reciprocated.[42]

Orenstein also found that sex is put first before the relationship has even started; intimacy and love are expected to follow—rather than sex being a result of developed affection.[43] Alcohol, she says, plays a big role, adding to the depersonalization. The combination of drinking and casual sex is nothing new, but now it's a "signal" that the hookup doesn't mean anything.[44] People have sex, not because they're attracted to each other, but because of the effects of alcohol.[45] This explains the Tinder mentality of picking through a pile of partners just to have drinks and sex. Attraction isn't really needed—alcohol acts as a blinder, for the eyes and the soul.

Given all these factors, trends in sexual activity over the past several decades aren't looking good. Overexposure, oversexualization, depersonalization, and pornography have desensitized us to sex. Either we've grown cold in our attachments or we don't become attached at all. We move from one sexual partner to another without ever connecting with anyone and without exploring who they are as individuals. We're overindulged but never satisfied. We're grasping for something, anything, to make us feel alive and to drive away the despair that dampens our spirits, but none of it works because we're not getting what we really need. Instead of finding happiness that comes from living a full, sensual, connected life, we're desensitized and lonelier than ever. We're lost in a sea of plastic images, ill-formed desires, and detached relationships. We're adrift in the loneliness of it all, and we're drowning.

CHAPTER 8

Becoming Sexual Experts

As soon as a person becomes an object of appetite for another,
all motives of moral relationship cease to function, because as an
object of appetite for another, a person becomes a thing.

IMMANUEL KANT

People call it "making a connection." Anyone who's had the experience of making a connection knows that it is the best thing that can happen in a romantic encounter. These days it is possible to meet someone, to be attracted to them, to feel the roots of your hair heat up and a flush to your face, to go to bed with them, but to still never know them. All of the interactions and movements that are necessary to get from zero to sex can somehow skate over the surface, leaving the depths of that person unexplored and unknown. You are as physically close to someone as it is possible to be, but somehow you never touch—not really.

That kind of sex *can* be fun, but it always feels disposable. Even when it's fun, you never really take leave of yourself or learn anything new. It can also, more often, leave you feeling worse: more solipsistic, more confined in your thoughts, more aware of your distance from everyone else. The objective in a romantic encounter should always be to break through the barriers and escape yourself for a while, to *discover someone else,* to find a whole new universe in another thinking feeling person. Each one of us is, as Erich Fromm wrote, "a unique entity, a cosmos by itself."[1] And by opening ourselves up to someone else, we can also discover new depths within ourselves.

The recognition of another person and their separateness from us is part of the mystery of love. But the way we relate to each other in modern life makes this harder. Instead we are encouraged to treat other people as a means to an end, and not as an end in themselves. We are encouraged to use people. In sex, we are encouraged to use our sexual partners for our own sexual gratification and never to look past this to the person beyond. When we do this, we turn them into an object, but we also ensnare ourselves in a trap of loneliness, where we have only our own thoughts for company.

Pamela

I have experienced this objectification in my life. A lover might have seen me naked before we had sex, and he has an image and expectation in his mind. He thinks he knows what I want sexually. He makes assumptions about me. I have been with men who have already had their minds made up about what they were going to do with me. Sometimes I sense a calculated energy in the way they behave toward me, and that can be quite intimidating— and disappointing.

The objectification moves in the other direction too. Men often feel the pressure to objectify themselves and feel like they have to live up to all the hype they're building, but they don't. No woman wants that. It's always better to get to know and discover what that person likes, to try to break through and make a connection. It can happen quickly if you are authentically in tune with that person: "love at first sight!" But it can also be part of a gradual process. The common elements are that there needs to be a genuine connection and the heated, euphoric recognition of attraction in a real other person.

These days, because so many people assume they know who and what I am
before they meet me, I often don't get the chance to start at the beginning,
to be that naive, young girl who is curious and who wants to dance the
intimate, fun dance of romance. But that thrill of adventure and discovery
is what makes sex interesting, not having premeditated mechanical sex based
on someone else's solipsistic fantasy, or some formulaic blueprint for how a
romantic encounter should happen.

Each one of us isn't made to be like everyone else. Every woman is
different, just as every man is different, and true eroticism is getting to
know each as they are. We shouldn't be judged by a standard established
by past sexual experiences or a sexualized culture. If we do that, our ideals of what's desirable will become very limited based on whatever society
deems "the perfect woman" or "the perfect man." When you allow outside
things to determine desirability, a person becomes an object onto which
you project your already formulated desires. But women (and men) aren't
a blank canvas where a man can transcribe another woman's image. She's a
complete painting all her own, full of unique detail, washes of blues, reds,
and yellows, deep shadows and wide-open spaces. A man becomes a great
lover by growing in knowledge of *her*, the individual—a subject of desire
to be known and embraced, not an object to be used as a tool to execute a
pornographic or collective ideal.

When an external model, whatever it might be, becomes the source
of knowledge and information about sex and sexuality rather than the
woman herself, she is removed from the picture—and she feels it. She
feels the distance. She feels the depersonalization. She knows the pain of
having others imposed on her. This is particularly hurtful when the source
of knowledge is pornography. As Rae Langton wrote in *Sexual Solipsism*,
"At first, an encounter with pornography is a way of imagining being with
a woman. Later, an encounter with a woman becomes a way of imagining

being with pornography.... Why choose to have one's imagination and relationships invaded, and made to march to an alien drum?"[2]

The same is true for men. As women are pushed and pulled into an overly sexualized, pornographic culture, they are seeing men through the gauzy film of erotica instead of getting to know each man in his own uniqueness, as the sexy individual he actually is. A woman saturated in this kind of contrived eroticism fails to focus on her husband or partner— his own body, the spirit behind his eyes, what excites him, how he moves, and the way he touches her face, trailing his calloused fingers down her neck. Instead, in her mind, she sees the image of a man with another face and another body doing things the man she's with doesn't enjoy. Neither women nor men want to be judged by an objective standard. They don't want to be an *other*; they want to be seen, known, and desired as *themselves*. In sex, both individuals need to be fully present, together in their hearts and minds, without the intrusion of celluloid specters or haunting memories.

Objectification, like overexposure, kills sex. When we typically talk about objectification, we put it in terms of instrumentality and denial of a person's full humanity; they're reduced to their physical body without having spiritual or emotional significance. The sexual revolution didn't solve this problem of objectification. It broadened it by making sex itself *objective* instead of *subjective*. When the sexual revolution overexposed sex, it became categorical not personal. Sex was no longer between one man and one woman; it was between *men* and *women*. Men became experts on women, and women became experts on men. Our desires became informed by others, by generalized categories, by objective sources, not by another individual person.

When it comes to loving someone, we become incapable of rendering an objective evaluation. Parents who love their children are not experts on the cuteness of their children. They can't be. They love their children, and it's their love that determines how cute their children are. This is why a parent's evaluation of their child is a purely subjective experience. Sex is the same way. Was it good for you? Was it fulfilling for you? Those aren't objective questions. You can't render an objective answer based on past experiences, because sex is emotional. If you do that, it's your mind that's having sex, not your heart.

What the sexual revolution did by giving us so many sexual partners and overly exposing us to sex is it took a subject that was supposed to be influenced by emotion (which makes us incapable of rendering an objective evaluation) and made it a cerebral experience. The mind functions for only one purpose—to make rational comparisons and render judgments. It determines what you should and should not do by looking at evidence. Once you decide to have sex, your mind is supposed to turn off and run completely on emotions, fueled by animal impulse. That's why sex is called carnal. It's when we are our most primal selves. This is why it's so liberating. This is why dystopian literature like *1984* and *Brave New World* portrays an oppressed people as those who are controlled by totalitarian regimes that either ban sex altogether or remove all emotional connection from it. Sex equals individual freedom, and there is nothing so liberating in life than being set free in sex. When you join with another *real* person in that most primal moment of release, it's powerful.

That's one reason we're so drawn to it. We're free but not isolated because we're connected to another person who knows us and desires us. It's in sex that we are supposed to be our most natural selves. It is a deeply personal, emotional—and subjective—experience. But when we objectify it and evaluate it, according to external standards or past experiences, we deny ourselves freedom and connection. We become caged to the judgments and "expertise" of others based on information outside of ourselves.

Because of the sexual revolution, women are now being judged based on all the women a man has slept with or all the women he has seen in porn or entertainment. The same is true for men. These images, which inform and shape our desires, always come to mind even if it's subconsciously, causing us to judge our newest sexual partner. This creates an emotional disconnect, and it also causes a great deal of insecurity. If you're having sex with an "expert," someone who thinks of sex and evaluates *you* based on previously gathered knowledge that has nothing to do with you, then you will be intimidated and worried about your performance and appearance instead of intimacy and connection. The act will be reduced to physicality instead of emotionality. It will become an objective exercise instead of a subjective experience. In essence, it will become two "tools" having sex instead of two people making love. This is deeply unsatisfying and dehumanizing.

The sexual revolution posited that the more sexual exposure we experienced, the better lovers we would be. But, as we've seen, that's not true. Overexposure and multiple partners have driven us to gather knowledge about sex and men and women in general, making us experts—but we're not supposed to be experts at sex. Two people are supposed to experience sex together, figuring it all out in each other's arms and looking into each other's eyes. The "information" you gather is experiential and subjective. This shapes your desires for one another and no one else. You become excited by the other person's body, how she catches her breath when you touch her, the angle of his face when he turns his head, the way she moves her hips, the way he lifts you up, the feel of her breasts in your hands. No other comparisons or experiences should play a part. He is everything you want. She is all you desire. It's all about her—and it's all about him. It's about feeling and sensing, not thinking, calculating, or planning. It's heart centered, not mind oriented. It's sensual not sexual.

Every one of us wants to be treated like a human being, not an object to be used and judged. We're not a car you buy at the dealership. We can't be experts in other human beings. We can be experts when it comes to an object, with a car or a house. We can examine its functionality. Does it have air conditioning? Is the car automatic or manual? Is the house one story or two? Do these functions fit your goals? Human beings don't have these criteria. You can't say one woman's breasts are objectively perfect. The question is, do *you* think they're perfect? Do they excite you? You can't say one man's genital size is the right one. The question is, does he satisfy *you*? Do you desire *him*? This is a personal question, and no one else can answer it for you. There is no objective standard, and if you put one onto him, you have made him an object. You have judged him. You have reduced him and dehumanized him. You have made him a tool to be used to meet your objectively constructed desires—a means to an end. The goal of sex, then, becomes about sex itself, and sensual connection with another person is lost.

CHAPTER 9

Goal-Oriented Sex

Ejaculation is not orgasm, to give birth to children is not orgas-
mic. Orgasm is the involvement of the total body: mind, body,
soul, all together. You vibrate, your whole being vibrates, from
the toes to the head. You are no longer in control; existence has
taken possession of you.

INDIAN MYSTIC OSHO

Prior to the sexual revolution, sex was generally less goal-oriented and more intuitive. Beyond couplings that were arranged for familial or economic purposes, when a man met a woman, he was instinctively drawn to her. He felt immediate desire, and she responded without any objective standards dictating to her whether he was desirable or not. They were drawn to each other from an inner compulsion, and sex was the expression of that intuitive connection—desiring, needing to be desired, making love. It was a dance, and it never ended—the masculine and feminine, husband and wife, in a perpetual embrace, an encirclement of lustful desire and steadfast love.

The sexual revolution turned that dance into a quest for sex. Orgasm became the goal. Men, of course, have always been prone to this, but women, in the past, tempered that masculine intent with their feminine soulfulness and inward, circular approach to sex. This balance, however, has been lost. With the sexual revolution and the saturation of sex on the American psyche, sex became the objective for both men and women. Put bluntly, women embraced a more masculine approach to sex. This isn't an absolute, of course. Women intuitively want the goal to be a relationship, which is why they often futilely look for long-term partners within the hookup culture. But they still get swept up in material-mindedness and too often join in the rush to have sex, to give the man an orgasm even as they fake theirs, and then move on.

While orgasm is certainly an important part of sex, it can't be the goal. That's because it's only the physical part of sex. When we reduce love-making to sexual climax, we're just focusing on our bodies. We're disregarding the intimacy that leads up to it. We're flying past the other person in our race to the finish line. We're just using each other to masturbate and ejaculate. Sex becomes a push toward a final destination, not a journey of mutual exploration. There's no real joining of two people, no soulful intensity, because no one is completely present in the act.

What we need is a means-oriented sexuality that puts the relationship, not orgasm, as the goal—as with Tantra, sex without climax being the focus, sex where the hormonal buildup without release occurs, thereby stoking the fire of desire. Who said sex had to be about orgasm? What if sex is supposed to be about increasing desire—without an outlet? What if sex is supposed to be about embracing hunger? Erotic desire is supposed to fuel us. If we want sex to be deeply satisfying, we have to be bound together, body *and* soul. No wonder people today are becoming sexually numb—they're not tasting the full joys of sex. They're suffering from sexual myopia, which dulls sensitivity and quickly snuffs out the flames of desire.

For the man, once he has an orgasm, he's pretty much done. His interest in sex diminishes quickly. That's why a man can so easily roll over and go to sleep after he has climaxed. It's finished, his desire is quenched, and he isn't engaged any longer, not physically or even emotionally. His fire has gone out. This can be quite frustrating for the woman, especially if her own sexual needs have not been met. She's lying there, looking at him sleeping with her fires still burning. She hasn't been satisfied emotionally or physically. He didn't take the time or make love selflessly. Typically, women already take longer than men to achieve orgasm, so if a man is only concerned about his orgasm, they won't get much satisfaction out of the experience. Rabbi Shmuley points out that this is such an important part of a relationship that in the Jewish faith, a man is obligated to pleasure his wife sexually before he pleasures himself.

Given the high use of pornography in our society and how it creates insecurity due to objectification, one has to wonder if this isn't one of the reasons 40 percent of women suffer from sexual dysfunction.[1] There are others, of course, including biology, but according to researchers, self-image is a factor: "Women have higher body dissatisfaction than men, and it interferes with their sex life more," Jacqueline Howard writes in an article titled, "Who Orgasms Most and Least, and Why." "This can impact sexual satisfaction and ability to orgasm if people are focusing more on these concerns than on the sexual experience."[2] If a woman is worried about her appearance and the man fails to connect with her emotionally because he has other women floating in his head, sex won't be as enjoyable as it could be.

The better a woman feels about herself, the more relaxed she'll be having sex, and the more likely she'll have an orgasm—especially if the man takes the time to make that happen before he dies the "little death" and goes off to sleep. But if the man is only thinking about his pleasure and doesn't recognize the importance of spending time with his wife, sensually exploring her body, and giving her the attention she deserves, sex will become drudgery for her.

This leads to greater dissatisfaction in the overall relationship. Elisabeth Lloyd, a professor of biology and philosophy at Indiana University-Bloomington, observed that "Women who have better sexual relationships with their partners also have more satisfied relationships in general, and it improves the quality of their relationships. So in general, a better sex life leads to a better relationship, which leads to a better sex life. It's kind of circular."[3]

If a woman isn't enjoying sex with her partner because he's too fixated on his own orgasm, the relationship will suffer. The whole point of sex has been lost—that it's about the dance, the two becoming one. It's about enriching the relationship. The woman needs to be satisfied as does the man, and both need more than physical gratification. For sex to be truly fulfilling, lovemaking needs to be a three-dimensional experience— physical, emotional, and spiritual. Ejaculation alone doesn't meet this need. It satiates the body, but not the heart and the soul. For all three to be satisfied, the couple needs to experience an emotional and spiritual orgasm as well.

We know what a physical orgasm is. It's the muscular contractions caused by external stimulation that leads to pleasurable release. It's body-centered. To have a physical orgasm, we don't even need another person. It can be done alone or with a tool. It doesn't matter. The material orgasm is simply a physical response and doesn't generate any sort of emotional or spiritual connection. This is the orgasm that has become the goal in American society. Once it's achieved, many people think that's all there is to lovemaking, but this goal-oriented sex undermines intimate connection.

To have that connection, another kind of orgasm must be experienced: the emotional orgasm, and it requires another person to be present, not just physically but emotionally. Together you enter a higher state of awareness as you experience powerful sensations brought to life by joining your bodies and minds. Light, color, touch, and sound—everything is brighter and more intense as you're pulled out of yourself and into the comforting, exhilarating presence of another person.

This opens you to an even deeper connection as you become attached to the spirit of another, something that is most profoundly experienced in marriage. The spiritual orgasm takes you to even greater heights because it is soul-centered. It leaves the physical behind. You're no longer aware of your body. You become part of everything around you and the person you love in one ecstatic moment. This mystical joining can't be experienced alone or with someone you're not close to—it can only happen when you know someone intimately. Together, as the husband and wife gaze into each other's eyes, they experience hypnotic engagement. Joining together in this spiritual ecstasy, they experience emotional vulnerability, a greater spiritual awareness, and even, in some cases, mystical vision.

This is the kind of lovemaking that quenches our desires. This is what satisfies our souls. If we were making love like this, imagine how our relationships would change. If sex could be transformed from a mere physical act to an energized, rapturous, and healing experience, wouldn't couples long to be together instead of putting off sex as if it were a chore? Wouldn't sex be so much more satisfying? And, wouldn't the result be happier, richer, and longer lasting relationships?

When we make love like this, we become human again, not just part of the machine, isolated and alone. We connect with another person, spirit on spirit. We're set free. The spirit is lifted from the body, the finite meeting the infinite. In that one electrifying moment, we are completely focused on each other. The world falls away, and we touch eternity. We breathe life into each other. Everything else disappears. The noise. The clicks of technology. The synthetic trappings. The voices of the crowd. Even time disappears. Only two people remain, wholly present, fully alive, joined together as one.

This orgasm is not just inward, in which we focus solely on our own pleasure, thoughts, and fantasies. It's an outward orgasm that unites us with another person. We're thinking not about our own pleasure, but another's. In that moment, we are complete. The feminine and the masculine, undivided.

When we stop treating sex (the physical orgasm) as the goal and approach it as a means to spiritual connection, sex will meet our most fundamental need—to be known and loved. The epidemic of loneliness that plagues us will vanish. Out of all human experiences, only the orgasm has the power to connect a man and a woman spiritually as their bodies join. Only in this moment are two people merged physically and spiritually. In the midst of carnality, sex is also deeply spiritual. This is why the marital bond is so intense and carries with it a power unlike any other relationship—it satisfies our desire to connect with another spirit.

Sex that brings together mind, body, and soul makes us want more of it, because it's so fulfilling. Our hunger will be for that one person who makes us feel alive, and we will return over and over again to be filled. There, in those arms, gazing into those eyes, tasting those lips, we will find wholeness—reenergized, transformed, and unchained from the heavy weight of a lonely world.

CHAPTER 10

Eating Ourselves to Death

We are hungry for more; if we do not consciously pursue the More,
we create less for ourselves and make it more difficult to experience
More in life.

JUDITH WRIGHT

We live in a consumer-driven culture that promises to give us everything we desire. If we have an itch, we scratch it, an urge, we satisfy it. If we can't, we complain because we think we're entitled to it. We show signs of being an overindulged, spoiled, satiated society that has forgotten what it's like to go hungry, to feel the pangs of unmet desires. Everything is at our fingertips. If we want something, we go to the Internet and we're sure to find it.

We're always feeding because we're hungry, but we're not being satisfied. We're focusing on our lesser appetites, stuffing ourselves full of material possessions, entertainment, distractions, and disconnected sex. But these don't nourish us. They leave us empty as soon as we've consumed them.

Pamela

I have several friends who gave themselves over to sex in the sixties, and now they say they regret it. The orgies, the stream of sex partners whose faces they can't remember—it all meant nothing. They tell me how they regret their broken marriages and missed opportunities. Now, in the twilight of their years, they're alone.

Indulgence was synonymous with the sexual revolution. Satisfy every craving. Express every emotion. Gratify every lust. Gone were the days of prudish reserve, suppressing our desires, waiting for the right person, delaying gratification. We had been set free. No longer would we be plagued by hunger. Restraint made us uncomfortable; now comfort is the goal. Why feel the pain of waiting for the right person? Why experience anxiety when you can purge it with ongoing sex? Why let the pangs of yearning build until that moment on your wedding night when you see a woman's body for the first time? Why spend time trying to rekindle desire for your husband when you can satisfy your sexual longings with another man? Quench your desires and numb your senses until you don't feel anything.

In the midst of this demand for comfort, our pornographic, oversexualized culture has primed us for sex. We're constantly titillated. Everywhere we turn, there's sex. We're in a continuous state of foreplay, the flames of desire being constantly stoked. The songs we listen to seduce us. The books we read, more sex. The way we talk to one another—our language is drenched in sexual innuendo. Even the news is about sex. We see it everywhere. It sinks into us. The greed of sex drives us to consume. We long for release, and the culture of instant gratification is right there, urging us on. You want sex? Have it. You don't have to look far. Turn on the computer. Scan a dating app. Hook up with a friend. Sleep with a coworker. It's all there, ready to be consumed.

The irony is that this cultural mindset has left us more uncomfortable

and less satisfied than ever. That's because we're not meant to gratify every desire or tickle every sexual fancy. We're not made for fleeting
pleasures—sleeping with one person after another, having an affair, turning on porn to slake our thirst. Even masturbation can lessen our sexual
yearning for our loving partner, who should serve as our principal sexual
outlet. We're made to sink our teeth into something that lasts. Distractions are cheap perfume. The sweet smell quickly turns sour. We need to
slow down, exercise restraint, and let our hunger linger.

If we don't allow ourselves to feel hungry, we won't realize what we
really need. Snacking all day is a deception. The salty bags of chips, the
sugary candies don't nourish. We're not hungry, but we're not thriving
either. We've become desensitized to our own needs. It's only when we
eat a wholesome meal that we'll feel alive again. That's when our bodies
are strong, our minds clear, our hearts light, and our spirits free. Our
hunger drives us toward these better things. We need to let it. If we
embrace our hunger, we'll achieve more and fly higher, because we'll be
using that energy to reach our goals instead of just feeding our lusts. Our
hunger will drive us vertically toward the greatest hunger of all—the
desire for spirituality. This is the goal of sex—to be *spiritually* connected
to another person. Sexual desire stems from this deep need for completion
and oneness. It purges us of loneliness—physically, emotionally, and spiritually. The hunger and ravenous desires we feel correspond with each kind
of loneliness, and we need to be aware of all three if we're ever going to
be fully satisfied.

When we are physically lonely, we feel detached from everyone around
us. Physical desire can only be met by material things. Sometimes that's
a person, but it can be anything—watching porn and erotic films, reading erotic novels, having sex with friends, and having sex with strangers. It doesn't matter. It's physical, and if our goal in sex is to feed our
bodies, then this is the only desire we'll satisfy. And we'll do it over and
over again. If sex isn't available, we'll look for other things to fill the

void—cars, houses, clothes, electronics, and entertainment. You name it, we'll consume it.

The materialism of our culture keeps us locked in this loneliness. We want something more, but we just don't know what it is. We feel desire, we feed it, we have sex, we buy things, we devour more and more, but then we crash. The pain is still there. The loneliness hangs over us like a shadow. We feel that ache even after we've slept with someone new every day of the week and even as we sit in front of a screen dulling our senses with pornography.

Another kind of loneliness is not feeling needed and loved. We can be in the middle of a crowd and still feel lonely because no one values us. We don't feel significant. It's as if we could disappear, and no one would care. We look out across the sea of faces, but we don't see any looking back at us, needing us. We are alone. We've connected with people physically, but our hearts remain caged within, untouched, isolated.

All the material goods in the world won't fill this emptiness. We need more. Our emotional desire drives us to find someone who will put us at the center of his or her world. We have a mental and psychological desire for the polar opposite—the masculine or feminine—that pulls us out of ourselves and toward another. But as exhilarating as this is, a spiritual loneliness still plagues us. We feel as if no one understands us, no one sees us for who we are. While it is important to be alone sometimes and to understand and appreciate solitude, loneliness is more about not being recognized for who you are. The most rewarding relationships in life are those involving someone who knows the real you.

Pamela

After reading my poetry, an actor friend told me, shaking his head, "You are the most famous unknown person in the world. Nobody knows you." It's moments like this that dispel the alienation that often comes with fame.

Not being known—this spiritual loneliness—fuels spiritual desire. We feel the hunger in our souls—to be known, to have the shadows fall away from our faces, every detail seen and understood. Only God, of course, can know us completely, but we're not in perfect communion with him. As long as we live in this world, we need another person to complete us, to join with us and know us.

When we join with another in this way, the loneliness fades. Our hunger is fed with the nourishment it needs. But it doesn't end there. It's a lifelong journey to know and be known. Our physical desires, our emotional needs, our spiritual longing to be known isn't fulfilled in a day, a year, or even ten years. We are ever changing and growing, and our spirits are eternal. We go through different life stages, our bodies get older, and we change over the years as we gain new experiences, meet new people, learn new things, overcome challenging obstacles, suffer losses, and celebrate victories. When we have someone go through each stage of life with us, needing us, knowing us like no other, keeping that desire alive while at the same time satisfying it, we are complete and we are never lonely.

This is the longing, the hunger, of every human being. We want to be loved. It's the human story, a theme woven through every tale from every land, but we keep getting lost in the telling of it. We confuse sex with love, material with spiritual, things with people. We walk in shadows instead of light, alone instead of with the one who loves us. We drink only when it rains, never diving into lakes of fresh water where the sun glistens on the waves. But that can change. We can experience passion that is anchored to intimacy, the two tied together in a sensual embrace. We can feel those warm waters close around us as if we're one with every drop. We can feel alive again, the blood beneath our skin quickening at our lover's touch, every part of us hungering for more, our body flushed from our faces to our toes. The days when we foraged among the thorns and thistles can come to an end, and we can begin tasting the grains of the fields and fruits of the orchards. We can satisfy our hunger. We can be filled with love.

Part Three

THE FEMININE EROTIC MIND

CHAPTER 11

Captured by Desire

He knew that when he kissed this girl, and forever wed his unutterable visions to her perishable breath, his mind would never romp again like the mind of God. So he waited, listening for a moment longer to the tuning fork that had been struck upon a star. Then he kissed her. At his lips' touch she blossomed like a flower and the incarnation was complete.

F. SCOTT FITZGERALD

There is no one way to be a woman. This is a major lesson of modern feminism. It's everywhere—in the pages of lifestyle magazines and *The New York Times*, Twitter timelines and Tumblr posts. Feminism is now very much in vogue, and the message it has brought to the mainstream is that women should consider themselves free from the trappings, norms, and strictures of a male-dominated society.

Pamela

I believe in the maxim, "No rules!" Nobody should tell women how to behave or dress or live or love. It is up to each woman to decide what is right for herself. Women should be free to be themselves, not bound by sexism, which women still experience even with all the successes of feminism. I certainly

have, and I've learned to overcome it. I've been on the receiving end of quite
a lot of sexism during my life. Before I began modeling, I was a shy, quiet girl
who did not know how to handle fame and too often found myself trying to
be accommodating, going along with the demands of others. Later I learned
to stand up for myself, to make my own choices, and to define myself on my
own terms, not those of others. I am proud of being able to be tough and
independent-minded when I need to be, which is why I'm a fierce advocate of
the idea that there is no one way to be a woman.

However, if that message is to mean anything, it must be taken seriously,
and we're not sure the type of feminism that enjoys popularity today really
does that. It's wonderful that women today are celebrated and encouraged to
choose their own path. Women should be free to defy conventional ways of
behaving, speaking, and dressing. But—and this is important—they should
not be made to feel as if they must do so. That is also telling women what
to do.

There is considerable pressure on women these days from a mainstream
culture that claims to be feminist to discard traditional notions of femininity and sexiness. Women today are encouraged to reject the classical
ideals of romantic love and to make themselves available sexually without commitment. This is often seen as the progressive "modern" lifestyle.
Women who don't do this, who prefer to conduct their love lives in an
"old-fashioned" way, can often be made to feel as if they are behind the
times, or even as if they are "betraying" feminism. The institution of marriage, or even of long-term monogamy with a man, is often dismissed as
an outmoded holdover from a patriarchal past, and we have sometimes
heard women say that it demeans women to get married or to enjoy relationships with men.

We think this goes too far. Rabbi Shmuley believes a woman's identity
as a woman is inseparable from femininity and from the classical ideal of

the complementary relationship between the sexes. We both think it's good to throw out inequalities between men and women, but we also think there are plenty of differences in relationships that are important to keep.

Pamela

I have always wanted to feel feminine, to be treated with dignity for who I am—as a woman. And for me, this is intrinsically connected to romantic love, being desired, being loved and chosen by a man. It's a fundamental part of my identity as a woman, and that is just as valid as any other identity. I, or any woman, should not be made to feel less of a feminist or less of a woman for wanting to be loved in this way. And while I'm not telling any other woman how she should behave, I believe there are many women who feel, as I do, uncomfortable with the pressures put on them to give up on true love. There are many women who feel undervalued and lonely and even exploited in the modern "sexual marketplace" where they are expected to be out for themselves. There are many women just like me who long for a relationship of equals but opposites twin travelers on the path to old age.

Every major relationship I've had in my life has confirmed that these needs are at the core of my identity as a woman. I reject a "feminism" that tells me this is an illegitimate part of my experience, or that I am somehow wrong about my own feelings, or that I am being a bad woman for being faithful to myself. The sexuality of men and women often expresses itself differently, and I'm fine with that. I live for that.

Thinking back to the start of one of the great romances in my life, I couldn't tell you much about what was happening around me. All I remember is he moved across the room, his eyes fixed on mine, and then my face cupped in his hands. He wanted me, only me. At that moment, the fire was lit. He chased me all the way to Mexico and didn't give up until I married him. I couldn't resist. I didn't want to. He captured me with his desire, and I never wanted to be without it.

That moment burned into my heart. His desire ignited mine, and from those flames, love was born—my soul mate, even though, much later, life and circumstances beyond our control took their toll on our marriage. Relationships can and do end, but none of that takes away from the fundamental rightness of that original feeling—the reason we all go in search of love. After all these years, after the pain, the heartache, and struggle, I can still feel that moment when his desire awakened mine, the passionate energy that bound us together. I live for that experience—to be wanted, desired. For me, this is a central longing and drive of womanhood—to be the center of a man's world where no one else can take my place.

Sigmund Freud once wrote, "The great question that has never been answered and which I have not yet been able to answer, despite my thirty years of research into the feminine soul, is 'What does a woman want?'" Every woman is different, of course, and there isn't one single recipe for how women can be happy and fulfilled in love and life. However, while it might be difficult to provide *the* answer, *an* answer can be provided. The answer offered here specifically addresses women in or seeking heterosexual relationships—there's no assumption to speak for women (or men) in LGBT relationships. Everyone should be afforded the chance to see if this is the answer that suits him or her.

From both of our experiences, the answer to Freud's question is that a woman wants to be *chosen*. She wants to be the one and only. She wants a man to fix his eyes only on her as his own. She wants to be the feminine that joins with his masculine, the *yin* to his *yang*, the Shakti to his Shiva. She wants to be the sun around whom his planet revolves and in whose light he basks. Only she can satisfy the yearnings of his masculine soul.

This might come as a surprise to those who have always heard that a woman wants unconditional love and protection. As mentioned earlier in the book, if a woman wants only unconditional love and security in a relationship, she would be content with her parents' love. She's not. That's because her parents didn't *choose* her. She's their child and they love her unconditionally. They would love her whether she was distinguished or not. But a man *chooses* to love her, confirming that she is special. His love isn't as certain or secure as a parent's love, but she still wants it even though he could leave her. He could cheat on her. He could divorce her. Why would a woman leave the security of her parents' love to risk the insecurity of a man's? Because she wants to be chosen, set apart, desired above all others, not just physically, but emotionally and spiritually. She wants it more than anything, and she will endure struggles, losses, and hardships, as long as she knows her husband adores her.

Rabbi Shmuley

I have spoken to many women who tell me this is what they want most in a relationship—to be desired. One woman I counseled struggled greatly in her marriage because she wasn't the center of her husband's world like she needed to be. There were a lot of reasons for this—neglect isn't always the result of the husband purposely being selfish. In this case, the husband withdrew from her because of his own struggles. He had suffered setback after setback professionally—something that can be very emasculating. He invested a lot of money on a venture and lost it. Then he became ill with testicular cancer. After that, he changed. He became very withdrawn. Very quiet. He felt like a failure. He was able to get a new job, but he still wasn't the same. He no longer expressed any interest or deep desire for his wife. At times he barely spoke to her. He continued to be a great father but not a great husband because he felt emasculated.

His wife began to distance herself from him, and it became a vicious cycle because he wasn't meeting her core need to be desired. She told him she didn't care about the money and she understood his health issues, but it was no excuse for how he was treating her. *"I'm the one being punished,"* she said. *"I'm the one being denied. I'm working hard, taking care of the kids, working two jobs, and all that is fine, but I need to feel like I'm the center of your life. I don't feel that way, and it makes everything else so hard. I can do without money and things as long as I feel like you are really focused on me and nourishing me as a woman. That's all I want."*

Her husband responded by saying he couldn't give her what she needed. She was asking for too much. But was she? She simply wanted to be desired by her husband. In a marriage, you don't get emotionally involved when you feel like it. It takes work and commitment. Marriage is about connection, irrespective of circumstance. It's not about desiring a woman only when you feel masculine— to the contrary. Sometimes, it's when a man doesn't feel masculine, when he feels like a failure, that he needs to remember what's truly valuable, and it's not his job, how he feels about his manhood, or how much money he has in the bank. It's about the woman he loves. This man's wife needed to feel desired, and her husband wasn't making her feel that way. He was despondent because he felt emasculated, but if he had treated her like a woman, he would have felt more masculine. By giving his wife what she needed, it would have gone a long way to restoring his sense of manhood. That's the beauty of the dance—the masculine and feminine, both giving and receiving, building each other up to be what they're meant to be.

Unfortunately, this couple eventually divorced. She ended up marrying a man who wasn't a professional big shot, but he doted on her, adored her, and that made her happy. Did this make her selfish? Does a woman's need to be desired, to be special, make her narcissistic? No, not at all. We all feel this way—men and women. We just express it in different ways. We need to know we're valuable and not replaceable, that we have significance. This is natural and good—it's part of being human. When we deny it or when it's neglected, we feel like we're not living to our fullest, that we are somehow less than we should be.

One of the reasons we're so unhappy in this materialistic culture is that we feel replaceable, interchangeable, as if all of our uniqueness has been reduced to our physical contribution. It's one of the reasons we distract ourselves with overindulgence and material accumulations. We don't feel significant because we base our value on what *we do* instead of *who we are*. We're consumed with doing instead of simply being. In truth, none of us wants to be desired merely for what we do. We think that's what we want, which is why we spend so much time and energy building careers and trying to be successful. But we know, deep down, it's not enough. It's transient. It won't last. All of our successes can disappear. We can be replaced at work. Our talents can fade. We can lose our abilities. We can lose our wealth. If our specialness is based on what we do, we won't be so special because it can be gone in an instant.

This is why we're growing increasingly anxious and unhappy. We think we're just like everybody else or worse. We don't feel good about ourselves; we don't feel valued—just another shadow stretched across the landscape of life. Our insecurities are magnified by a superficial, materialistic culture that measures our worth based on our accomplishments. We're always comparing ourselves to what others do and what they have, instead of focusing on who we are as unique individuals. This heightens our insecurity and lessens our confidence.

To be truly secure, we need someone in our lives to think we're intrinsically extraordinary—imperfections and all. Ultimately, for many, that someone is God, but we need it from people too, and most importantly from the person who can truly complete us. When a man chooses a woman simply because of who she is, not because of what she does for him or anyone else, she feels a deep, soothing joy, and her heart answers his because he sees her as special—the one out of the many. It's irresistible. There's no one else but her, no competition, no comparisons. This makes her feel secure in his love—a restful state of being that is deeply satisfying and uplifting.

This theme of being chosen is woven throughout history and literature, in cultures all over the world, from the Hebrew Scriptures, to the legends of courtly love in Europe, to sacred stories told by Native Americans across the sea. In the Scriptures, God chooses the nation of Israel from all others, setting his love upon them as his special people, comparing their covenantal relationship to that of a husband and his bride: "For your Maker is your husband—the Lord Almighty is His name—the Holy One of Israel is your Redeemer; He is called the God of all the earth."[1] The security of this love is unwavering as God promises his chosen people to be faithful to them forever: "I will betroth you in righteousness and justice, in love and compassion. I will betroth you in faithfulness, and you will acknowledge the Lord."[2] Israel responds with gratefulness and adoration as they are elevated above all other nations in God's sight.

This longing to be chosen, to be set apart from all others, is reflected in the stories of many cultures, showing how it is a common thread that ties all of humanity together. One such story is a Lakota myth called the "Love Flute."[3] It's the tale of a quiet young man who sees a beautiful girl and falls in love with her. She's his heart's desire. He thinks about her from sunup to sundown. She's all he wants, but he's too shy to speak to her. One day, he leaves the camp, his heart heavy with discouragement. He shoots arrows into the sky, and magically they linger in the air, pointing forward. He follows them, and they lead him to a forest where he meets two Elk men. The men give him a flute made of cedar, with holes formed by a woodpecker's beak. All the animals helped make the flute, and their voices sing with it. It's infused with life, power, and passion. The Elk men tell the young man that when he returns to camp and plays the flute, the animals will sing with him. The music will speak to the girl for him, telling her of his love and desire.[4]

When the young man returns to the camp, he plays the flute. Its music attracts every girl there, and they come out to see who's playing. But one girl hears the music and knows it's speaking only to her—she's the one the young man desires. Drawn to him, she leaves her home and walks out of the camp to join him on a hill where she listens to him play, her heart opened by his passion and love.[5]

This is what every woman wants—to be chosen from all others, to have music played only for her, stirring her soul. Some might think this suggestion makes a woman too dependent on a man for her happiness. Is a woman dependent on a man for happiness? Is her sexuality defined by his? Does the feminine really need the masculine? These are questions any self-respecting, sexually liberal culture will no doubt ask, and they need to be answered if this suggestion is to be taken seriously.

To begin with, we are not saying a woman should subjugate herself to a man. Less so are we saying that women require men for fulfillment. Women are individuals. They can find happiness, purpose, and fulfillment outside of a relationship. But both men and women are *more* fulfilled in a relationship. And a man should meet a woman's needs as much as she meets his. Responding to his desire isn't catering to him or giving him power—the power is also the woman's because she can refuse to answer his call, and he's left holding a boom-box over his head hoping she'll change her mind.

Neither are we saying a woman is dependent on a man for her identity and purpose in life. She is perfectly capable of providing for herself, expressing her individuality, understanding who she is as a woman, and succeeding in a career and contributing to a community just as a man does. She can be happy without a man, depending on what she wants in life. Some women choose to remain single, and they're perfectly content with that choice. They want to focus on work, service, or other interests. Some women don't desire men, and instead enter loving sexual relationships with other women, and those relationships can happily and fruitfully function according to a different dynamic. Regardless of the path a person takes, we all need to fill the loneliness within our souls. Most of us meet that need in marriage or long-term relationships. In saying this, we're not reviving female oppression but restoring a balance between the masculine and the feminine and passionately connecting the two as one.

Throughout human history, this balance has been lost, rediscovered, and lost again. Most of the time, the feminine has been oppressed by the masculine. Women have been reduced to their functionality as mothers or sexual objects, labeled as irrational and incapable, and even denied expression of their powerful sexual impulses. In the past, women were considered to be less rational than men, emotionally fragile and prone to passion or "hysteria"—temptresses and vixens who captured men in webs of manipulation and cunning. In the West, elements of Christian religious thought saw a woman's sexuality and passion as a threat that needed to be controlled. Some patriarchal cultures severely oppressed women, covering them to hide their sexuality, selling them as child brides like slaves, mutilating their genitals to "keep them faithful," and treating them as a man's property instead of independent, equal, and free human beings—practices that have continued in Islamist societies to this day.

In the eighteenth century, the belief that women should be controlled took a different slant in the West. Women were still seen as emotional beings who were sensually impressionable, but they were placed in a more protective frame and kept from the coarse and vulgar facets of society. They became delicate flowers carefully arranged in a proper vase. Strict moral codes developed to protect women from exposure to sexual immorality. They couldn't go to the theater, for example, because their minds were too impressionable. Over the years, as women were denied exposure to expressions of sexuality, they began to be seen as passionless. Cold and aloof. Any sign of overt sexuality by a woman was considered immoral and even pathological. If she was interested in sex, she was diagnosed as a nymphomaniac.

This view of women changed in the twentieth century as research in human sexuality, particularly Alfred Kinsey's *Sexual Behavior in the Human Male* and *Sexual Behavior in the Human Female*, found that women were just as sexual as men. The walls that caged female sexuality were crumbling. Women pushed their way through toward sexual liberation. No longer would they be virgins or sluts, Madonnas or whores. No longer would their passions be controlled. They were meant to be free to express their sexuality as fervently as men. Former stereotypes and categorizations fell away, and over time, female sexuality showed itself to be more multifaceted than patriarchal Western civilization ever imagined.

Pamela

Discovering the many facets of one's own sexuality—and the freedom that comes with that—is a journey. Before I was a model, I was painfully shy. It was an awful, debilitating feeling. I was always my own worst critic. Nobody cared as much as I did about my flaws or my body. When I began to model with Playboy, I started to push myself to the limits and broke through that shyness. This was when I started to become aware of the liberating sensuality that was available to me. I experimented with it, and I realized I could have walked naked down the street and nobody would have cared. I realized that everyone else was more concerned about themselves than they were with me. I didn't need to live in bondage to how other people saw—or didn't see—me. Why did society tell me I had to be so covered up anyway, or remain a prisoner to fears about how I look?

For me, transcending this shyness helped me notice the beauty in others too—all the shapes, sizes, and unique qualities of other women. It's a mosaic of beauty. Sexy and free. When we are so preoccupied with ourselves, we're not really looking around us. I believe women need to be brave to discover themselves and have fun with their sexuality—then their personal life and how they look will be fine.

Part of that discovery is to see that there is more than one dimension to their sexuality. Meredith Chivers, a highly respected researcher in human sexuality, came to see just how multifaceted a woman's sexual nature really is when she performed studies to analyze the differences between male and female sexuality.[6] In one landmark experiment, she measured physical sexual responses of men and women as they looked at sexual and nonsexual images and asked them to record which ones aroused them. By examining both their physical, objective responses, and their cognitive, subjective responses, Chivers believed she would get a better, more objective picture of what men and women desire. The images were varied, including men with men, heterosexual coupling, women with women, people walking and doing exercises, and even animals mating. After analyzing all the data, Chivers concluded that men and women are essentially different in how they respond sexually.[7]

The women, both gay and straight, were physically aroused to one degree or another by all sexual images, including apes mating. Their cognitive responses, however, didn't match their physical responses. The straight women said they were mentally aroused by heterosexual couples having sex, and the lesbians said they were aroused by women. None of them said they were aroused by animals mating or women exercising. As reported by Daniel Bergner in *The New York Times*, Chivers observed that "with the women, especially the straight women, mind and genitals seemed scarcely to belong to the same person."[8]

The men, on the other hand, measured no disconnect between their minds and bodies. Heterosexual men were physically aroused by images of women and men together, as well as women with women. But they had no physical arousal when they saw only men together. The reverse was true for homosexuals; they had no interest in images of women. None of the men were aroused in any way by the apes mating, neither physically nor cognitively. To determine whether or not this could be a nature-versus-nurture issue, with environment influencing sexuality, the same experiment was done on men who had transitioned to female. The transgender women had responses consistent with men, not women. Their brains corresponded with the arousal of their biological male sex.[9]

As we can see, the adage that men will have sex at any time with any person doesn't quite ring true. It seems women are the ones who are sexually omnivorous—at least physically. This, of course, doesn't mean women actually want to have sex at any time with any person. Otherwise, as Chivers said, women would want to have sex—and we're sorry for sounding ridiculous here, but we're referring to the research—with monkeys, and they'd all be bisexual in their orientation. That's clearly not the case, but this does show that a woman's sexuality is much more complex than a man's.[10]

After analyzing the data, Chivers speculated that the seat of desire for a woman is in the mind, not the body.[11] Men are aroused by what they cognitively and physically desire, but for a woman, her body's response doesn't involve actual desire. That's because the female body is always in a state of readiness, not because she always *wants* to have sex but because her body is always *able* to have sex whether she desires it or not. This state of receptivity puts women in a vulnerable position because she can be forced to have sex. It's theorized that to protect her from harm, a woman's body automatically begins to lubricate the vagina whenever anything sexual is perceived; this involuntary physiological response protects women when penetration occurs. It's purely biological—a physiological protection mechanism.[12]

Because of this, we can't look to a woman's body to determine her sexual interest. We have to look to her mind—that's where the connection is made. Chivers explains that a woman's "reflexive physiological arousal," along with her mind being the "domain of lust," makes her desire "more receptive than aggressive":[13]

> One of the things I think about is the dyad formed by men and women. Certainly women are very sexual and have the capacity to be even more sexual than men, but one possibility is that instead of it being a go-out-there-and-get-it kind of sexuality, it's more of a reactive process. If you have this dyad, and one part is pumped full of testosterone, is more interested in risk taking, is probably more aggressive, you've got a very strong motivational force. It wouldn't make sense to have another similar force. You need something complementary. And I've often thought that there is something really powerful for women's sexuality about being desired. That receptivity element.[14]

Marta Meana, a researcher who serves on the board of *Archives of Sexual Behavior* with Chivers, agrees that a woman's desire is cognitive.[15] Women, she says, want to be "the object of erotic admiration and sexual need."[16] A woman's erotic fantasies, compared to a man's, "center less on giving pleasure and more on getting it."[17] This insight reveals the intensity and passion so many women want. It also illustrates the contradictions inherent in female desire. "Women want a caveman and caring," Meana says.[18] They want intensity and intimacy. Strength and gentleness. This can be confusing to a man because she sends mixed signals, but she's consistent in her contradictions. The man brave enough to hold these contradictions in balance has unlocked the secret to the female erotic mind.

This contradictory nature is part of the mystery and complexity of the feminine. The man who forces a woman into one mold or the other reduces her and himself because he doesn't benefit from the fullness of her femininity. To love and desire a woman is to fearlessly know and embrace her extraordinary nature, the fire and the water, the depths and the heights, the passion and the intimacy, her body and her soul. She is more than she appears, and a man needs to pay attention, see her many facets, to satisfy her.

CHAPTER 12

Erotic Fantasy

So sweet and delicious do I become,
when I am in bed with a man
who, I sense, loves and enjoys me,
that the pleasure I bring excels all delight,
so the knot of love, however tight
it seemed before, is tied tighter still.

VERONICA FRANCO

One of the great tragedies of the sexual revolution is the wedge that has been driven between masculinity and femininity. This modern era could be characterized as the great divorce between these two polarities. Femininity has gone one way, and masculinity has gone another. They've become equal, but separate. When they do meet, there's often discord, not harmony. In some instances, no distinctions are made between the two. Femininity and masculinity as biological or psychological constructs are denied or fused into a single entity, and an androgyny begins to take their place. The result has acted as a solvent on heterosexual relationships and has created a culture riddled with isolation and loneliness. Try as we might to deny human nature, the masculine and feminine are distinct yet dependent on each other—one aggressive, the other receptive. Without the union of these two energies, we're incomplete.

For us to understand what a woman wants, we have to understand both the feminine and masculine and their relationship to each other. There's a reason nearly 70 percent of women say they want their partners to take the initiative with them sexually.[1] They want to feel the intensity of being chosen. They want to feel seductive, magnetic, and desirable.[2] They want a man to take control; they want to feel the intensity of masculine strength as it meets the power of feminine assent. Women want the chase; they want to be sought and won over. They might be politically correct in other areas of their lives, but when it comes to the bedroom, they want a proverbial bone through their hair and a strong man lifting them up and carrying them off to the cave.

When it comes to sex, female fantasy can be downright primal. A woman wants a man to make her knees weak, to seduce her with his powerful presence. She wants to experience a man's sexual strength. She wants to feel the intensity of the polarity between her receptive femininity and his masculinity. It's important, however, to distinguish here between male initiative and sexual coercion. No woman wants to be coerced into sex. Sex without consent is rape, and rape is one of the most heinous crimes imaginable. No woman would ever desire to be physically forced into sex, and no man should ever get the false impression that "no means yes," or that women want to be sexually manipulated and controlled. The scourge of rape in our time is a catastrophe, which causes untold suffering to millions of women.

While no woman wants to be violated, women do want, within the confines of a consensual and loving relationship, to be sought after, to be wooed by men who desire them, to be in a position to accept or reject male attention. Male initiative places the woman in a position of power, and it is in assuming this power—the power to choose—that feminine sexuality thrives.

Strength is one of the hallmarks of masculinity, and the feminine is attracted to its power like a magnet. One theory that accounts for this is derived from evolutionary psychology—a woman is attracted to the strongest man because she needs his protection to survive. Women aren't living in caves any longer, and they can protect themselves, but the instinct—so the theory goes—is there. This primal urge is integral to feminine sexuality. Despite human progress, feminism, and modernity, a woman is still drawn to vibrant masculinity. The more she feels a man's strength, the more feminine she feels—and feeling feminine is beautiful. A woman is happiest when she is authentically herself, and a man's masculine energy excites and affirms that part of her. He makes her feel like a woman.

A woman's sexuality is intense, and she needs intense desire to fuel it. When women don't have it, many will attempt to get it vicariously, through sexual fantasies, erotica, and porn. They might have an emotional connection with their partners, but there's no passion. Well-worn familiarity, mutual support, and gentleness aren't enough. They're important, but women need passion along with connectedness. They need fire, not just tender words and soft touches. They need the masculine to meet their feminine, which means men need to embrace their masculinity, express it, and bring it into the sexual relationship. These polar opposites must be present for there to be sparks.

Researcher Marta Meana found this to be true when she was working with women who suffer from a condition that makes intercourse physically excruciating. Increased desire, she found, correlates with less painful sex.[3] But the way to increase desire has "little to do with building better relationships" and simply being intimate.[4] Being sensitive and saying tender things like "Is this okay?" during sex isn't appealing, she found.[5] It does nothing to arouse desire. It's loving, but there's no oomph, she told Daniel Bergner, author of What Do Women Want?[6] "Female desire," Meana said, "is not governed by the relational factors that, we like to think, rule women's sexuality as opposed to men's."[7] Good, loving, empathetic relationships don't guarantee desire. Hugging, kissing, and snuggling are great, but if that's all you have, you're out of balance. You have a lot of feminine energy, but where's the masculine? Without it, the relationship becomes dull and boring.

RABBI SHMULEY

Men often don't get this because, first, with the passage of time desire diminishes in relationships, and second, lust has been demonized in our time. This is especially true in religious circles. If you tell a husband he should lust after his wife, he recoils. "But that would be wrong!" he says. "You're supposed to love your wife, not lust after her." The tenth commandment says that a man should not lust after his neighbor's wife, which means, by direct implication, he sure ought to be lusting after his own! He should desire his wife, not just spiritually, but physically. It's not sinful. It's natural, and a woman needs more than a nice, considerate man. She wants passion. She wants her husband to lose control, possessed with wild abandon ignited by her desirability.

When this essential element is missing from their relationship, many women wander, either in their imaginations or tragically in reality. I have seen this many times, women who contact me for counseling because they're having an affair or about to have one because passion is missing from their marriage.

A school teacher came to me once because she was having an affair with a colleague at work. She had started talking with the man innocently enough, but then the conversations became more sexual. The more they talked, the more sexually explicit and forthright he became. He said things to her that were right out of her fantasies. He knew she wasn't being physically fulfilled at home, and he gave her what she needed. She didn't understand how this man could know her better than her own husband. The relationship turned into a full-blown affair because he had tapped into her erotic imagination and met a legitimate, deep-seated need. The woman was surprised by her own actions because she didn't understand herself, and her husband didn't either.

How many men are baffled when their wives suddenly tell them they're leaving them, or when they discover their wives have had a passionate love affair? They don't understand. They've loved their wives. They've provided for them. They're good fathers, faithful husbands—everything they should be. They even go on dates with their wives and pick up groceries on the way home from work. They shuffle the kids from one place to another. Why isn't it enough? What went wrong? The honest truth is it isn't enough. Women want masculine energy igniting their own feminine fires. They want passion.

Regardless of how a couple works together to build a life—going to work, raising children, taking care of the practicalities of life—when it comes to an erotic relationship, a woman wants the erotic fantasy. She wants to be seduced by a man. Too often men complain that their wives are turning them down when they try to become intimate, but chances are, most of the time, they're not acting like admirers who are wooing their wives, but husbands who simply expect their needs to get met. They also assume that a woman merely wants to be cared for and loved, failing to see that she wants him to lust after her. The way into a woman's bed is not through love alone, but through desire fueled by love, and love fueled by desire.

CHAPTER 13

Passionate Connectedness

I love you more than my own skin and even though you don't love me the same way, you love me anyways, don't you? And if you don't, I'll always have the hope that you do, and I'm satisfied with that. Love me a little. I adore you.

FRIDA KAHLO

RABBI SHMULEY

A woman came to counseling and said, *"Rabbi Shmuley, my husband just doesn't get me."* She was a very accomplished woman, smart, and a law professor. She was a moral woman with good values, and she and her husband had one child. He was a good provider for both of them and a decent, upstanding man, but she was depressed because he was completely distracted and traveling constantly. When he was home, their relationship was "acceptably affectionate," but he didn't seem like he really desired her. *"Some of my male colleagues are attracted to me,"* she said. *"They behave respectfully, but I can still see that they're attracted to me. How can they want me, but my own husband doesn't?"*

I met with the husband separately, and the man admitted he had lost interest in his wife. *"I have to be honest,"* the husband said. *"I'm*

just not that into my wife. I love her, I want to see her happy, we have
sex regularly, and my purpose in having sex is to pleasure her, but I'm
just not attracted to her. I get almost nothing from the experience."

When I met with both of them together, I asked the wife to tell her husband what's wrong. She looked at me and said, *"He just doesn't get it. He doesn't get that a woman needs to be adored, that she wants to be wanted, that she wants to feel desired all the time. She needs to feel special. I feel very ordinary in our marriage. I feel like he doesn't really want to know me. When I get undressed at night, it's not like he stares at me with desire in his eyes. I feel like my core need is not being addressed. That core need isn't being provided for. My core need is to be desired, cherished, and adored. I want someone who wants to be with me. I feel sometimes like my husband doesn't even miss me."*

The husband responded by saying her demands were unreasonable. *"You want too much of me,"* he fired back. *"I work hard for you and our daughter, but it's not enough. We have a regular sex life, and I make sure you climax. I give you gifts, but nothing seems to make you happy. You complain all the time, constantly critical. That's off-putting, and it's one of the reasons I'm not really into you."*

She shook her head, *"No, the opposite is true. A woman knows when a man is really into her, and you don't get it. You don't understand what my real needs are. My real need is to feel that you are irresistibly drawn to me. I see that from other men, but I want it from you. I want it from my husband, but you're not giving it to me."*

Many women in America are living in a sensual desert just like this woman. They might be having sex, but it's unsatisfying. They're not experiencing the passion they long for, and it's making them feel dispirited and discouraged. They look in the mirror and see lines on their faces and dullness in their eyes. They remember when they felt alive, when their husband's touch electrified them. But now there's only distance, and when they are together, there's emptiness between them. They wonder if they'll ever feel that excitement again. What happened to the passion? Where's the intensity?

Pamela

In every marriage, it's important to achieve balance between the caring and the romantic. Rabbi Shmuley's anecdote describes a loving relationship that has lost its passion. On the other hand, I caution that it's important not to undervalue the loving side of a relationship. This is the kind of love that U. A. Fanthorpe described in her poem "Atlas": "maintenance is the sensible side of love."[1]

Make no mistake, this is an important side of love—it is the part of love that gives us understanding and unconditional support for each other. It is the part of love that accepts each other's flaws and forgives them and that's happy to muddle along when things are not going well. It is the kind of love that sees something comforting and magnificent in standing together for a time before death parts us, the kind of love that gives us meaning in our lives. But it is not all of love. It must exist in a balance with passion, movement, and mystery, the elements that give it immediacy and exhilaration, or it will slowly die down or breed resentment.

Women need someone to pay attention to them, to connect with them both physically and emotionally. It can't be one or the other. It has to be both—naked body and naked soul. If she's only a naked body, she feels objectified, exposed, disconnected, used. If she's only a naked soul, she has a friend but not a lover. She's drinking the water, but there's no flame to keep her warm. She needs both, and she needs a man who will bridge these two parts of her feminine sexuality with masculine desire. She wants passion, but she also wants intimacy.

"A woman has tremendous powers when the dual aspects of psyche are consciously recognized and beheld as a unit; held together rather than held apart," Clarissa Pinkola Estés writes in *Women Who Run with the Wolves*. "The power of Two is very strong and neither side of the duality should be neglected. They need be fed equally, for together they bring an uncanny power to the individual."[2]

Breanne Fahs, a clinical psychologist who specializes in sexuality, interviewed forty women over three years and found desire for connection to be a major theme running through all descriptions of their best sexual experiences. Her interviews revealed "stories of intense, textured, and tangible pleasure" full of "emotional connection."[3] The best sex was when their partners were *attentive*, and they experienced "intense physical pleasure along with *embodiment*, where they felt fully present."[4] For many, this intensity and emotional attentiveness were more important than physical pleasure,[5] and sex without it made them feel empty.[6]

No wonder so many women are dissatisfied with their sex lives and relationships. They want passion *and* connectedness, but they're only getting one or the other. They go through the day feeling bored. They pick the kids up from school, and they're bored. They go to work, and once the business of the day is done, they still feel bored. They sit beside their husband as he watches sports on television, and they feel like they're disappearing, sinking into the sofa, unimportant, insignificant. They have sex, but there's no electricity between them, no presence, and no deep desire. She gets up and cleans her face, the loneliness washing over her like the water dripping from her cheeks. This is why 69 percent of divorces are initiated by women[7]—many don't feel desired by their husbands. The passionate connection they once had has been broken, and they're adrift in the relationship.

This seems to be happening more in marriage relationships than non-marital couplings.[8] Women and men break up at the same rate when they're not married, but in marriage, it's the women who are out the door first. The big difference, we believe, is the level of intensity and how it's maintained. In nonmarried relationships, the man is still wooing, still choosing, still making the woman feel special. There's still a sense of unavailability, mystery, and forbiddenness—all of which fuel desire. But in marriage, the choosing has been signed and sealed. The man often thinks he's done his job and he can kick back and enjoy the peace and comfort of a complacent relationship. His wife has a ring on her finger. She knows she's the one, so why does he have to continue to make her feel special? But that's exactly what she needs. She needs her husband to continue choosing, desiring, romancing, wooing, and making her feel like she is the one. She needs that passionate connection and affirmation. Some think it can't be done in marriage, but we believe it can.

Too often, that connection begins to loosen as soon as the honeymoon is over, and the husband and wife drift apart. They begin to sense something's wrong, but they don't know what it is. The woman will say things like, "I'm just not happy, he doesn't understand me, we don't talk anymore, and he doesn't pay me any attention." But what she really means is "He doesn't desire me anymore, he doesn't make me feel special." When she tries to reach for that connection and he doesn't give it, she shuts down. Just a little at first, but the more it happens, the more she shuts down. Then one day she realizes how lonely she is. There's a gulf between them, and she doesn't even know how it got there. She wants to feel alive again. She wants to be wooed and romanced and treated like a lady. She wants her knight in shining armor to fight for her hand. She wants to be desired. When she doesn't get it, the loneliness becomes overwhelming and she either cheats or leaves.

Too many marriages slip into this dull, platonic pattern and fail to keep the passion burning. They choose intimacy but forget the passion. They choose sex, but forget the sensuality. They make love to the body but not the spirit. They fail to keep the balance of both. The body needs to be cherished, held, wanted, and desired. The soul needs intimacy. If you don't give to the body, you're bored. If you don't give to the soul, you're lonely. James Laughlin paints a picture of this balance of intimacy and passion in his poem "Oh Best of All Nights, Return and Return Again." [9]

Sex and passion are the things in a relationship that remind you that this is another person, "different from you, together with you." When passion goes out of a relationship, when it slowly slides into domesticity and the mundane everyday, we easily forget that we are two different people, apart but together. Functioning as one unit for so long—buying the groceries, driving the kids around, keeping schedules—our individual personalities start to disappear into the routines of married life. We become automatic, practiced, like clockwork. Sameness swallows our sense of newness and mystery. Our sexuality slowly disappears into sameness too. Libido dies from familiarity. The lust and attraction that bring two people together come from the differences between us. It is a common saying: "opposites attract." In a real sense couples are opposites, feminine and masculine, and that is why they are attracted to each other—this difference can't be forgotten or the intensity in the relationship will fade.

Attraction pulls us together, but it dies when we coalesce, losing our distance from one another. When we forget our differences, when we begin to collapse into the same person, we lose the thing that attracts us to each other in the first place. That is why it is bad for a relationship to forget real sexual passion—the essential counterweight to the more mundane, comfortable side of love. A healthy relationship is held in tension. It is a union, but between two separate beings, not two bodies with one soul. To keep our relationships and marriages alive, we must be careful to maintain our independence from each other—and that is the best way we can respect each other. As Kahlil Gibran wrote: "Give your hearts, but not into each other's keeping. For only the hand of Life can contain your hearts. And stand together yet not too near together: For the pillars of the temple stand apart, And the oak tree and the cypress grow not in each other's shadow."[10]

Most Americans think they have to choose one or the other—passion or intimacy. Some women even joke that they wish they had two husbands, one for the bedroom, and the other for the rest of the house. They don't think they can have both in one man. But they can have both—a lover and a friend, romance and companionship, the flame and water. But how? They seem contradictory. Won't the water put out the flame? Won't the flame consume the water? How do we keep both going? How do we reconcile these two opposites? Is it even possible?

A sensual revolution in our sex lives is the solution to this dilemma, because it is *passionate connectedness*. In sex, we connect only through the body. It's about doing. Sensuality is sharing. We don't abandon sexuality for sensuality, but we use sexuality to create sensuality. Sex, desire, and passion create deeper connectedness. Our passion leads us to become soul mates, and our intimacy feeds our passion. It's circular, and we keep the circle going with desire.

CHAPTER 14

Give a Woman What She Wants

A gentleman holds my hand. A man pulls my hair. A soul-mate will do both.

ALESSANDRA TORRE

F or men, it's hard to figure out many women because they're full of contradictions—and that's not a bad thing. A woman wants passion and intimacy. She wants someone safe, but a bad boy. She wants sex and sensual connection. She wants a man to explore her body and connect with her soul. The man who can bridge all these contradictions with fiery desire, who can respect a woman's differences instead of trying to control or change her, will win a woman's heart and hold it forever.

Unfortunately, many men don't do this. They get married and the desire turns cold. The husband falls asleep in front of the television, never touching his wife, or he's scrolling through the computer, while she's alone upstairs. The months pass and they seldom have sex. Dullness enters their relationship. Some women in sexless relationships feel like they're dying a little bit every day.

Rabbi Shmuley

I am simply astonished by how many couples come to see me ostensibly because they are struggling with everyday conflicts, like not agreeing on how to discipline the kids, only to discover in counseling that they haven't had sex in months or even years. Most often it's the wife who reveals this detail and who seems to truly mourn the sexual death of the marriage. One couple I knew hadn't had sex in three years! The wife was in her late thirties. She and her husband shared a bed, but he might as well have been sleeping in the guest room. He was a public figure, and he was busy with work. She told me in a private session that she had been having thoughts about cheating. She didn't want to. She was horrified by the thought of her husband finding out. She didn't want a divorce, but she felt like she was wasting away. *"I need an affair just to make me feel alive again, to keep from drowning."* Fear alone made her refrain.

How many women are living this life? They look back to when they were single, and they wonder what happened to the vibrancy they once felt. Everything seemed to have turned gray. What happened to those days when her husband looked at her with hunger? Does this happen to everyone in marriage? Does everyone in a long-term relationship have to feel like they have one foot in the grave?

We don't believe they do, but for this to change, men and women need to learn how to passionately connect again. A man needs to be brave enough to desire a woman, and she needs to let him. To put it bluntly, this isn't happening because too many men are afraid of, and intimidated by, female eroticism. They want to tame it, suppress it, or neglect it. They don't want to invest the energy it takes to bridge a woman's contradictions, to keep passion alive while still remaining emotionally connected to her. After marriage, the man thinks he can just sit back and treat his wife like a passionless woman from the Victorian Era. He's turns her into a maid or a nanny to his children. He stops admiring her as a woman.

Women are powerfully erotic, and they want that intense sexuality to be met by the intensity of a man. For this to happen, men have to be strong. They have to be brave. They have to stop being lazy and spend time focusing on their wives, fulfilling her fantasies and desiring her as if it were the first day they met. Men get sidetracked because they are caught up in *doing*. They go to work, they care for the home, they run a business, they make money. They're always doing, doing, doing. But to love a woman, a man needs to learn how to *be* with her. He needs to open himself up to her and connect with her as a lover, not just a provider.

This tendency to treat women in long-term relationships as something other than a sexual being is what is driving men to have affairs, breaking hearts and destroying relationships. It's why pornography is becoming a substitute for a real woman. It's easier to turn on a computer than to take the time, to experience the vulnerability, and to put forth the energy to connect with a real, flesh-and-blood woman. It's easier to treat your wife like a co-worker who makes your life easier, and when you want hot sex, you turn to another woman.

A woman should never be forced to be either a saintly Madonna or a sultry Jezebel. She can be both in one person. This is the power of femininity. She can be a mother, a wife, and a successful CEO, but she can still be filled with passion and attracted to a man whose sexuality excites her. To meet that powerful libido, a man has to be brave. When he's not, he is sexually extinguishing his wife. Women are losing their sensuality that is altogether feminine, as men fail to passionately connect with them. Whether it's because of work, distraction from entertainment, fatigue, or desensitization due to porn, the result is the same: a woman's sexuality is being shut down. Her deeply sensual nature that cries out to be admired, chosen, touched, and known is dying.

One of the reasons for the sexual revolution was to put a stop to treating women as objects and tools. The days of women being reduced to their functionality were over—or so we thought. Today, too many women are still being treated functionally by men. No wonder marriages are suffering. Lazy men who thought that marriage could be put on auto-pilot stopped seeing their wives for the women they really are. They've neglected their wives' true selves—just as women sometimes neglect themselves, focusing on what they do instead of their inner spiritual and sensual needs.

Living and loving life in all its forms means knowing it, connecting with it, seeing it, feeling it, smelling it, tasting it. Life is sensual, not cold and mechanical. A woman's hair, the green of her eyes, the dimples when she smiles, the smell of her skin—these are part of her sensual nature. Her soul, her spirit, longs to be known, to share thoughts, ideas, and feelings—this is what it means to be human. It's the source of her creativity, humor, intelligence, and imagination. When women aren't living a sensual, passionately connected life, they feel extinguished. What they want is to be known in all their aspects of being, and loved accordingly. The words of Bryan Adams' love song "Have You Ever Really Loved A Woman" might seem trivial, but they're actually very true: "To understand her—You gotta know her deep inside."[1]

Most men would say they want to really love their wives and that they don't have any intention of neglecting them. They want a sexually vibrant woman. But do they really? Or do they just want safety and security, saving erotic engagements for someone on the side, either in real life or through technology? Do they truly want a vivacious woman they have to keep up with, or are they afraid to step up and be man enough to desire the woman he married? Maybe in the back of a man's mind is fear that he can't satisfy her, that he isn't enough, so he shuts down. She's married to him, so he doesn't need to be anxious. This is why women's sexuality has been historically suppressed. Men are too weak to handle it. The more they pull away from their wives and relegate them to a functional role, the better they feel because they don't have to worry about measuring up.

Even if they have sex with their wives, many don't connect with them emotionally. Intimacy is out of their comfort zone. They'd rather be doing than sharing. They run from emotional connection because they don't want to be exposed. Why sit on the sofa with your wife in your arms, gazing into her eyes and being emotionally vulnerable, when you can work on a project, watch a ball game, or go out with friends? You were willing to be open when you were chasing her, when you were trying to capture her, but now you caught her. She's secure, so why make the effort?

Why? This is the question many men need to ask, and the answer is always the same—because she's worth it, and she needs it. She's special. She's beautiful. She's powerfully erotic. Her mind is a universe to be probed. Her body is a wonder to be explored. Her soul is an ocean of possibilities. She deserves to be desired. Her feminine spirit seeks the masculine to experience the fullness of life.

Many men fail to meet that need because they're exhausted from challenges in other areas of life, especially at work. A man comes home, and he needs to rest. He wants to have ten to fifteen minutes of sex and then fall asleep. He doesn't want a vixen to pursue; he wants a wife to make him comfortable. The years go by like this, and then one day he looks at his wife and sees someone he's not into. She's dull and uninteresting. But let's be honest. It's very possible that he's the one who makes her feel that way. He has done nothing to excite her passion and to connect with her as a complete woman. He has extinguished her sexuality because he feels inadequate. The result is boredom.

To cultivate the relationship, they must spend time together. The man must be awake, aware, and interested in this amazing woman he has chosen to love. He must take the time to know her in every way, and essential to this knowing is the embrace of the dual nature of a woman's sexuality—her outward nature that is cool, calm, and takes care of the children, pursues her career, and addresses the needs of her husband. This is the civil, loving part that enjoys quiet intimacy and connection. And he needs to know her inward nature, the deep recesses of her femininity where the "wild woman" of ancient lore lives, longing for someone to pull her to the surface and embrace her feminine glory, a wild man who can meet her face to face, fearlessly and with equal bravery and equal passion.

"The outer being lives by the light of day and is easily observed," Estés writes. "She is often pragmatic, acculturated, and very human. The *criatura* [inward being], however, often travels to the surface from far away, often appearing and then as quickly disappearing, yet always leaving behind a feeling: something surprising, original, and knowing."[2]

When these beautiful, sensual facets of a woman are ignored, when she is not being known and desired for who she truly is, she is wounded. She isn't living authentically because part of her is being denied. She needs a man to see past the outward parts of her and peer deep inside, where her passions burn like roiling lava beneath the earth.

"When both sides of the dual nature are held close together in consciousness, they have tremendous power and cannot be broken," Estés writes. "This is the nature of the psychic duality, of twinning, the two aspects of woman's personality. By itself the more civilized self is fine . . . but somehow lonely. By itself, the wildish self is also fine, but wistful for relationship with the other. The loss of women's psychological, emotional, and spiritual powers comes from separating these two natures from one another and pretending one or the other no longer exists."[3]

Instead of hiding from a woman's powerful sensuality, men need to have the courage to embrace it. Instead of letting it die, nurture it. Women, too, need to be brave. They need to be willing to embrace and reveal both natures, the outward and the inward, the domesticated and the wild, the known and the mysterious. A woman needs to tell her partner not only what she wants, but also her deepest desires—and the two are not always the same.[4] Being vulnerable in this way is the advantage—and the wonder—of being in a loving, intimate, monogamous relationship. You can be who you are, and you are loved. And desired! When you experience this connection and this wholeness, vibrancy will flow into every area of your life. You'll be free of boredom and insecurity. The gray will disappear, and life will explode with color again.

Part Four

THE MASCULINE EROTIC MIND

CHAPTER 15

Needing To Be Needed

One of history's greatest romances is the marriage of Napoleon and Josephine. It was a turbulent relationship riddled with passion, infidelity, and jealousy. Napoleon's letters to his "sweet and incomparable Josephine"[1] were filled with adoration and painful insecurities. He often worried he had lost her affection, and he pressed her for reassurances, pouring out his heart and waiting with impatient anticipation for her letters, for promises that he was the only one and that they would be together again. Without her, part of him was missing. "My soul is in your body," he wrote, "and that day on which you change or cease to live will be my death-day."[2]

Napoleon, a powerful figure in history, was reduced to a beggar before the woman he loved. He had chosen her from all others, and he couldn't bear the thought of her needs being met in the arms of another man:

In your letter, dear, be sure to tell me that you are convinced that I love you more than it is possible to imagine; that you are persuaded that all my moments are consecrated to you; that to think of any other woman has never entered my head; they are all in my eyes without grace, wit, or beauty; that you, you alone, such as I see you, such as you are, can please me, and absorb all the faculties of my mind, that you have traversed its whole extent; that my heart has no recess into which you have not seen, my prowess, my spirit are all yours. . . . If you do not believe all this, if your soul is not convinced, penetrated by it, you grieve me, you do not love me. There is a magnetic fluid between

people who love one another. You know perfectly well that I could not brook a rival,
much less offer you one.[3]

After years of infidelity, running up debts, and failing to produce an heir, Josephine was set aside for another. Napoleon divorced her, and his new wife gave birth to a son the next year. Despite the divorce, Napoleon continued to hold Josephine in high esteem, though she was devastated by the divorce. Following her death, an acquaintance told Napoleon she died of a broken heart. "She loved me, didn't she?" he said sadly and hopefully. Being the center of her world meant everything to him, even in the midst of brokenness.

A modern myth about the masculine erotic mind is that it's fixated only on sex, that physical fulfillment is what a man needs principally in a relationship to make him happy. While it's true that a man's erotic nature is different from a woman's, the root of his erotic desire is emotional. He wants to be loved and *needed* by the woman he desires. He wants to be special. He wants to be the only one who can satisfy her needs and fulfill her sexual desires. He wants to be validated by her, not simply for what he does and what he produces, but for who he is. He needs to be fully known by the one person he is connected to spiritually, soul to soul. When he's not, he's lonely and depressed. He's in a state of brokenness, and he feels like a failure. Men, contrary to popular belief, are intimacy seekers.

A man needs to be the center of his lover's world, just as she needs to be the center of his. He wants be the one who gives her new experiences, to do things for her no one has ever done before. He wants to be needed and to bring out her fire. When he discovers that some other man has done that, he's deeply wounded. He's emasculated and depressed, because his most basic need has been violated.

Being needed is inextricably bound to feeling significant. When a man feels insignificant, a deep loneliness grips his soul. This was the very first pain experienced by the first man in the Garden of Eden. Adam had God and the ministering angels for company, but he had no one who *needed* him—there was no one to make him feel significant, no one to cherish his unique gifts as a man. Adam had angels all around him, but they didn't need him. He needed someone to make him feel necessary, essential. He had no one to lean on him, depend on him, or confide in him. If Adam were to die, no one would miss him. This is why God made woman—"a suitable helper for him" (Genesis 2:18).

This need to feel significant doesn't mean simply feeling useful in the practicalities of everyday life. It comes from within—in the spirit—to be connected and completed by another spirit, someone who understands you and your pain of loneliness, a fellow sojourner in this world who makes you feel essentially important for who you are—that your very being completes another. You are seen and appreciated for more than just what you actively produce. You are cherished and valued for being you. This is a spiritual need that goes beyond the physical—a need that can't be satisfied in a world focused solely on material things and physical gratification.

Unlike girls who are often judged by their passivity (what they look like), boys are judged by their activity. They're raised with a focus on what they do. Play sports. Produce in school. Get a job. Provide for the family. A man's masculinity is very much tied to how successful he is. His manhood is inseparable from his ability to produce and provide for others. He is, therefore, validated through achievement and his career. He's judged in the world by his actions, so he needs confirmation from the most important person in his life that what he does is worthy. And yet, he needs more than this from her—and only her, the one he has chosen. He needs to know he is worthy for who he is. In her presence, he wants to be, not do. *Doing* is exhausting and drains the soul. *Being* is healing and fills the spirit.

A man wants to be able to provide for his family. He wants to bring home the paycheck, build the deck, fix the car, and kill the spiders. But he also wants to be the only one who meets his lover's emotional, sexual, and spiritual needs. She longs to be desired, to embrace masculine strength, and to experience sensual connection; he wants to be the one who does that for her. He wants to be the only one who can scratch that erotic itch she has deep within. When she either doesn't validate him or is so independent that she treats him as if he's not integral to her life, he feels as if he doesn't matter, that he's insignificant. No one wants to feel that way. If they do, they'll withdraw, cheat, numb themselves with entertainment, or pour themselves into work. The man will live his life feeling unnecessary, and the woman will feel as if she's no longer desired. The space between them will grow until there's nothing left to draw them to each other.

In our American culture, we've grown hardened to the idea of true intimacy and romance between a man and woman and the necessary connectedness of the masculine and feminine. We've lost the sense of needing to be known and adored, but this need is essential to eroticism. It's the very core of masculine desire. When a man is truly appreciated for his being, his erotic mind is triggered. It's awakened and aroused by a deep connection that makes him feel complete and significant in this lonely world. Being known and needed touches the very depths of who we are and stokes the fiery passion that ignites our desires and makes us feel alive.

Understanding and recognizing this need to be needed is not always easy for a man, especially if he has been raised to believe showing emotions isn't masculine and vulnerability is only for girls. But this isn't true; it's merely an attitude that has been imposed on men from a culture fixated on gender norms. As clinical psychologist, Jill Weber, says, "Underneath this conditioning is a child who, just like you, wants to feel loved for who he is. He desires someone who can be okay with him even when he's not winning, producing or 'on top.' "[4]

Pamela

Bringing up two boys as a single mother, I knew I needed to understand male psychology as much as possible. I found some of the most important insights in the work of Jean Liedloff, who spent time with the Yequana people in the

Amazon rainforests. She argued that the Yequana had a lot to teach modern Westerners about childrearing. Their practices were much closer to those of prehistoric man and much more attuned to human nature as it evolved over millions of years. Human babies—just like any other infant animal—have innate needs and instincts that affect their development. If those needs are not met—for instance, if a mother does not carry her baby and involve him in her adult life—this leads to developmental and psychological issues in later life.

A man who was deprived of physical contact as a child will experience a gnawing absence all his life, a void he desperately tries to fill. Liedloff writes:

> We are disengaged from our human continuum at birth, left starving for experience in cots and prams, away from the stream of life. Parts of us remain infantile and cannot contribute positively to our lives as older children and adults. But we do not, we cannot, leave them behind. The want of in-arms experience remains alongside the development of mind and body, waiting to be fulfilled. We in civilization share certain ailments of the continuum. Self-hate and self-doubt are quite general among us, in varying degrees, depending upon how and when the complex of deprivations affected our inherited quali ties. The quest for in-arms experience, as the years pass and we grow up, takes on a great many forms. Loss of the essential condition of well-being that should have grown out of one's time in arms leads to searches and substitutions for it. Happiness ceases to be a normal condition of being alive, and becomes a goal. The goal is pursued in short- and long-term ways.[5]

I was fascinated by Liedloff's claim that in Western culture we are too controlling and have too little faith in our babies' sense of self-preservation.

Babies have innate instincts toward self-preservation that have evolved over millennia. In America we try to police our babies' behavior down to every tiny detail out of a fear that if we don't they will get themselves killed. Liedloff pointed out that Yequana mothers had not forgotten respect for the natural instincts of the child and did not approach childrearing with a tyrannical need to control their infants.

One of the oddest outcomes of loss of faith in the continuum is the ability of adults to make children run away from them. Nothing could be closer to the continuum heart of a baby than to stay close to his mother in unfamiliar territory. All our mammal relatives, and birds, reptiles and fish as well, are followed by their young, in whose clear interest it is to do so. A Yequana tot would not dream of straying from his mother on a forest trail, for she does not look behind to see whether he is following: she does not suggest that there is a choice to be made or that it is her job to keep them together: she only slows her pace to one he can maintain.[6]

Liedloff's insights explain a great deal about the behavior of men in Western culture. In a strange way, my quest to understand my boys better gave me an insight into all of the men in my life. Suddenly I understood that the listless emotional insecurity of one man, or the compulsive habits of another, went back to their earliest experiences. The deepest needs men have and their innate human nature became clearer to me. Understanding all of this as a woman is key to building a deep, lasting, passionate relationship.

Sociologist Rebecca Plante, who has done extensive studies on the culture of casual sex, has also found that men are more complex than society has let on when it comes to relationships: "While some guys do view sex and desire as one and the same, many others—even those in the early stages of a casual engagement—want someone they know and trust on a deeper level." Men, she says, need to be empowered to express their real needs—"To say, 'I actually like to know my partner. I like to be in a relationship with her. I like to be connected to her. That's what turns me on, more so than that she's attractive.' "[7]

Men want to have sex, there's no doubt about that, but they want and need so much more. They want sex to be a part of a deeper relationship. Plante quotes men who confirm this: "We want to say 'I love you' before you do . . . we want to race you to love, and win. We want to love you so much that when we see a pretty face we think it's less pretty than we would if we didn't love you."[8]

When a man feels needed just for being himself, he's empowered and feels more like a man—and he's more giving and loving. In former, more refined times, men where inspired to prove themselves worthy so a woman would want him and need him. This motivated him to keep coming back, over and over again, to woo her, to earn her trust. His focus was on her, on desiring her, and she returned his attentions by affirming that he was the one to meet her needs. This intimate, giving connection drives away narcissism, which is rampant in our modern society. Too many people are detached from their relationships, focusing on sex instead of sensuality, intimacy, and romance. This breeds selfishness and self-gratification. When this happens, women no longer feel special or chosen—they just feel used and neglected—and men no longer feel significant. They feel expendable. One man is no more important than the next guy. If that's how things are, why should men be motivated to love, give, and serve? Why even try to do anything for a woman—she doesn't care.

No one wants to live this way, even though many people do. If he's truly in love, a man will want to serve his partner. He will put her first instead of himself. He will give to her and make her happy. She will respond by showing him how much she needs him, and he will be even more motivated to make her happy. As John Gray wrote in *Men Are from Mars, Women Are from Venus,*

> *When a man is in love he is motivated to be the best he can be in order to serve others. When his heart is open, he feels so confident in himself that he is capable of making major changes. . . . He is suddenly released from the binding chains of being motivated for himself alone and becomes free to give to another, not for personal gain, but out of caring. He experiences his partner's fulfillment as if it were his own. He can easily endure any hardship to make her happy because her happiness makes him happy. His struggles become easier. He is energized with a higher purpose.*[9]

When a woman needs a man, his soul soars. Without her, he can't fly; his wings are broken. He needs her presence, her attention, her dependency on him as her soul mate. Everything else can disappear, but never her, not her touch, not her eyes fixed on him, not her words of encouragement, not even her laughter. Pablo Neruda puts this so beautifully in one of his most famous love poems, "Your Laughter."[10]

Interestingly, poet and Jungian psychoanalyst Clarissa Pinkola Estés makes the connection between a woman's laughter and her sexuality, which puts Neruda's poem in a whole new light. A woman's sexuality brings joy, laughter, and healing both to herself and her lover:

> *Laughter is a hidden side of women's sexuality; it is physical, elemental, passionate, vitalizing, and therefore arousing. It is a kind of sexuality that does not have a goal, as does genital arousal. It is a sexuality of joy, just for the moment, a true sensual love that flies free and lives and dies and lives again on its own energy. It is sacred because it is so healing. It is sensual for it awakens the body and the emotions. It is sexual because it is exciting and causes waves of pleasure. It is not one-dimensional, for laughter is something one shares with oneself as well as with many others. It is a woman's wildest sexuality.*[11]

A man needs these waves of pleasure washing over him, cleansing him. He wants to leave the rat race of life, of always proving himself by what he produces; he wants to find rest in a woman's wild sexuality and feel the joy of her sensuality. He needs her to see past his career, his bank account, his honey-do list, to something deeper; he needs her to see him simply as the man who loves her and treasures every aspect of her being. He wants her soul to reach out to his like a plant reaching for the rain and the sun. He wants to feed her, enliven her, give himself to her so she can thrive. This reaching, giving, and joining is sensual, not just sexual. It's healing. It's peace in the turbulence of life, when, as Walt Whitman writes, "amid the noises of coming and going, of drinking and oath and smutty jest, there we two, content, happy being together, speaking little, perhaps not a word."[12] To rest in being and in loving—this is what a man wants most of all.

CHAPTER 16

Masculine Duality

When you know what a man wants you know who he is, and how to move him.

GEORGE R. R. MARTIN

I n *Women Who Run with the Wolves*, Clarissa Pinkola Estés tells the tale of Manawee, a man who, with the help of his dog, must learn the names of two sisters before he can wed them. The fable, which is fraught with frustration, distractions, and difficulties as the man tries to solve the riddle, illustrates how he must understand and embrace a woman's duality to truly connect with her; he must learn her two names—the civilized, thoughtful, refined nature that is focused on *being*, and the wild, passionate, creative, instinctive, and powerfully sexual nature that is focused on *doing*.

This sensual joining can only happen when a man understands and embraces both of these powerful feminine forces, when he desires the woman he loves in her beautiful complexity instead of wanting her to be only one way (Madonna or Jezebel). If he fails to understand her or neglects, dominates, or even resents one side of her, their love withers because she isn't being allowed to develop as a complete person. "If a woman hides one side or favors one side too much, she lives a very lopsided life which does not give her access to her entire power," Estés writes. "This is not good. It is necessary to develop both sides."[1] The woman who feels no emotional connection in sex will withdraw into depression. The woman who never has her sexual desires ignited and is treated only as the wife and mother will wither in loneliness.

The same is true of a man. Take what we've just said about a woman and flip it around. Men have two sides to their sexuality as well—the internal, instinctive, emotional, and intuitive side that reflects his soulfulness, and the physical, linear, task-oriented, active side. Both are necessary for a man to be a man, both are powerful, and both must be loved by a woman for there to be intimate, passionate connection. The man whose partner never wants to have sex will be lonely, and the man who isn't appreciated for what he provides and produces, who is never truly seen and known for who he is, will be distraught.

To avoid this, a man must know and appreciate—for himself—his dual nature. The same is true of a woman. If neither knows who they are, if they have shut down one side or the other, how is their partner supposed to know them? How will they show the other what they need and desire? They both need to embrace their full, harmonious sexuality. When a woman is complete in her femininity and the man is complete in his masculinity, the relationship is no longer two dissonant keys being monotonously tapped over and over again; it becomes a glorious symphony.

In her story of Manawee, Estés gives us insight into the duality of a man by including a symbolic dog. The man is his natural self, his outer nature, and the dog represents his instinctive nature. It is this part that discovers the names of the women. The dog symbolizes a man's deeper, intuitive side, which is the only part of his masculine nature that can discover the corresponding part of a woman. It is in this deep knowing that they find a partner equal to themselves, soul to soul, body to body, and heart to heart.

The difficulty a man faces getting to this point is when he neglects or distorts one side of himself. He allows his dual masculine traits to run afoul of the balance they need, and this becomes disruptive. He neglects his need to accomplish, achieve, and meet a woman's powerful sexuality with bravery and strength, and in so doing places too much weight on his sensitive, soulful side. Or he neglects his soul and becomes a desensitized, destructive, macho, even sadistic masculine force. Both are destructive to our humanity and relationships.

When it comes to sex and what a man wants from a woman, men are naturally very different from women in how they think and act. Generalizations though they are, the male and female erotic minds are complementary, not one and the same. They express many similarities, but it is a mistake to think of them as identical. One of the primary differences is the inescapable masculine focus on physicality. The man connects first through his eyes and only later through his heart. For him arousal comes unbidden, without even thinking about it. He heats up quickly, expends his energies, and cools down immediately. Everything about outward masculine sexuality is active and responsive to external stimuli.

This focus on external stimuli is why men are more vulnerable to porn addiction. Pornography stimulates the physically oriented, visual aspect of male sexuality, providing a superficial high, but yielding no emotional rewards. It skims entirely across the surface of male sexuality, but it is easy for men to get stuck there, unable to progress to deeper and more meaningful connections with women. There's no creativity, no imagination, no spiritual connection with another person. Left to a porn addiction, the masculine erotic mind is numbed and distracted, and he learns bad habits that become more and more difficult to kick. It is understood by consumers of pornography that it is artificial, but to many men this does not matter because sexual arousal for them can be brought about by real sexual experiences or simulated ones alike. Porn addicts, however, are still missing out on the thing they most need from their erotic lives—passionate connectedness, sharing, and emotional intensity. All of these are neglected with pornography. Only one side of the masculine erotic mind is being satiated—the soul is being starved.

Even though men are aroused visually, this doesn't need to be a negative. One woman should be enough to *see*—all of her beauty explored. Her body, after all, is a wonderland! Discover its secrets, dive into its depths. One woman is all a man needs, especially if they both are less shy with one another and unafraid to laugh or fail—to really show each other who they are. If they're playful, doing thoughtful things out of kindness and love—in the bedroom and out—they will be satisfied with the love they have and not have to look elsewhere. If a man is *really looking at* the woman he is with, he will have no need of anyone else, and the lure of pornography won't cross his mind.

Sadly, this doesn't always happen. In the twenty-first century, because we have forgotten how to make love, much sex between couples remains externalized, creating conditions that make men more likely to go astray. This touches on another, related aspect of the masculine erotic mind—novelty. It is often said of men that they grow bored with their sexual partners after the novelty has worn off. Sex with one woman, so goes the cliché, isn't enough for a man. This is seen as the explanation for why men become adulterers—as their wives age they are driven to pursue newer, younger, more exotic women to satisfy their drive for sexual novelty. They live out the lyrics of Hozier's evocative song "Someone New": "And so I fall in love just a little ol' little bit every day with someone new . . . love with every stranger, the stranger the better." Hozier's song could be described as the anthem of seeking novelty—and the despair that goes with it.[2]

Today, men are thought to be instinctive womanizers, always dissatisfied with a single woman, always on the lookout for someone younger or more desirable, always looking past their wife for something new. They've bought into the belief that this is what it means to be a man. They think to be the partner of just one woman for their whole life will make them feel incomplete, like a failure, as if they're missing out on what life should really be about: having sex with lots of women, being drawn to them simply because they pay them the slightest attention, but making no real connection. In the end, they wind up corrupting the women instead of cherishing them.

Men are seen as the natural adulterers, and it is even thought that adultery is less culpable in a man because he can't help it—that it's his nature. This is doubly sexist, because it holds women to higher standards of sexual fidelity, and yet it also diminishes men and removes their agency. These prejudices about male sexuality have become so ingrained that some scientists have even tried to invent scientific justifications for them. It's common to see the argument in evolutionary psychology that men are naturally unfaithful and long for a polygamous state because evolution has made them that way. In human prehistory—so the argument goes—men who had as many children as they could with as many women as possible became the ancestors of the next generation and passed on their unfaithful nature in this way. Generation after generation, this was reinforced, so that it is now built into the male psychology and can't be escaped. According to this view, the classical ideal of marriage is simply hostile to male sexuality: men will invariably be unhappy in a monogamous relationship. Men are genetically incapable of being satisfied with what they have and must be involved in constant sexual conquest to feel happy.

Even if all of this were true of the way men *do* behave, it isn't how they *should* behave. What's missing is the fact that men are conscious agents not automatons. They're spiritual—made in the image of God—not merely physical. They're rational, with the power of thought and reflection. They're not driven solely by their animal appetites. They have choice and agency, and they are capable of using it. In the Book of Job, Elihu calls his listeners, "Men of understanding"—they can employ their minds and not just give into their impulses. "Let us choose what is right; let us know among ourselves what is good."[3]

Being a slave to genetic programming and sin is just that: slavery. It is a state of subordination and unhappiness. Even when a man is driven away from his spouse by a feeling of incompleteness, he will not find completeness no matter how many women he sleeps with. It will not satisfy his existential hunger. Instead, it will only cheapen his sexual experience and perpetuate his longing. No sooner will he have slept with one woman than he will be lusting after the next, and if he is not careful he will find himself in a cycle of addiction and despair.

This search for someone new is just a side effect of the overstimulation of the physical side of the male erotic mind and an understimulation of the deeper, passionate, soulful side. A much healthier alternative is to be found in a passionate, connected sexual relationship, where the endless depth of his partner's soul opens up to him, and there is novelty enough for him to explore for a whole life. Without this, without looking inward for novelty, he will become bored, and the physical side of his sexuality will lead him to seek it in a dead end: in an endless succession of partners, none of whom truly satisfies him.

Real completion can only be found by recognizing that men are more than evolutionary machines acting on the level of stimulus and response. True happiness in love can only flourish when a man is complete in himself, living by both sides of his nature—physically and spiritually, naturally and instinctively, intellectually and poetically. There is more to men than just the need for carnal conquest. A man has physical needs, but he also has existential needs: the need to share existence with another so he doesn't feel so alone.

Mere sexual gratification cannot address a man's need for a substantive, sensual connection with another person. He needs a different kind of sex, built on a sturdier foundation. His whole being must be satisfied, not just his carnal desire. What a man needs most of all is recognition—emotional and physical connection within a romantic relationship—and to feel that he is the center of a woman's life. When he feels this, sex within marriage will be all the sex he needs. Here, in the embrace of enduring reciprocal passion, is where true male sexual fulfillment is to be found, not in an endless succession of temporary partners. One person can be all he needs. Love is more powerful than the impulse for someone new. A man can get all the novelty he needs from one woman, experiencing new things together, deepening love through spending time discovering new thoughts, new dreams, new ways of seeing the world through the eyes of the one he loves.

Another way this errant desire for novelty can manifest itself in men is by driving them to push boundaries, to compel a woman to do and try things she never has before. It must be said that trying new things is not always a bad thing—sexual exploration within a mutually supportive, committed, consensual, respectful sexual relationship is a good thing and is to be advised! It's something secret and powerful between two people. Pushing limits can be good sexually—and you can always say no! But when the impulse to push limits comes about as a result of the neglect of the emotional side of the masculine erotic mind—when it comes about because of the absence of passionate connectedness—it can become unbalanced, decadent, and even malignant.

The darker side of male sexuality is the need to conquer, to overcome, and, in its most decadent form, to corrupt. This can lead to disconnected sexual behavior, where the man pushes a woman past her natural boundaries, treating her body as a means to his own gratification, ignoring when she is uncomfortable. Indeed, it may be her very discomfort that arouses him. We see this in art and literature, from Don Juan and Casanova to William Hogarth's series of paintings, *A Rake's Progress*. The rake jilts lovers and corrupts virtuous women, stripping them of innocence to fuel the flames of his masculine desires. We find this rakish behavior depicted in Pierre Choderlos de Laclos' novel *Dangerous Liaisons*:

I shall possess this woman; I shall steal her from the husband who profanes her: I will even dare ravish her from the God whom she adores. What delight, to be in turns the object and the victor of her remorse! Far be it from me to destroy the prejudices which sway her mind! They will add to my happiness and my triumph. Let her believe in virtue, and sacrifice it to me; let the idea of falling terrify her, without preventing her fall; and may she, shaken by a thousand terrors, forget them, vanquish them only in my arms.[4]

Pushing boundaries can sometimes go too far, but we all have our fantasies, and it's incredible when you feel comfortable enough with one other person to share them. A man needs these moments when he can let go and feel in control, when he has a woman's complete attention—and holding a woman's attention is very attractive to a man. It's seductive to him because it taps into his inner sexual needs. He ultimately wants to be the only one who can satisfy her. He needs her femininity to draw out his masculinity so he can feel complete. He needs her to *see* him for the simple man he is—underneath all the external layers of expectation and achievement. The competitive world drains him, and he needs her attentions and occasional sexual (and consensual) "compliance" to refill him.

Sometimes he is so deprived of this, or so insatiable in his need, he'll even gravitate to a woman who is merely pretending her attentions. The prostitute who gives him exactly what he wants and lets him leave his work at the bedroom door. The secretary who doesn't challenge every decision he makes. The waitress who looks into his eyes every day at lunch and actually listens to him. These women are giving him something that touches him in the deepest possible way. Even if it's fleeting, even if it's not real, even if the woman ultimately just wants his money, the man will be drawn to it because in that fleeting moment of focused attention, he will be captured.

Of course, concentrated attention is very intense, and two people can't do it indefinitely. A woman can't constantly focus her attention on her man just to ensure that he is faithful—that would be impossible. It is also completely unnecessary. A man doesn't need the unbroken attention and relentless fawning of a partner. That would be exhausting for him too, because it demands his emotional reciprocation. But what he does need is a true connection in those moments when he is closest to his wife or partner. It is made all the more meaningful and sensual for him if it isn't all day, everyday. A little, but not too much; scarcity is important.

Pamela

This is why it's so good to spend time apart, to miss each other. Striking the right balance—keeping a sexual relationship in equilibrium—is the key to keeping a man interested and a relationship alive. It's important to keep things a little mysterious, a little sacred, and to ensure that, even in a monogamous relationship, sexual connection is not taken for granted. This isn't manipulation. It's the honest raw dance between two people who have separate lives that can come together and be interesting for each other—and fun. Sex is adventurous and exciting, even funny, as we get lost in each other. It's exploring and learning.

It's easy to see, though, how monogamy is so difficult, given the delicate interplay between the feminine and masculine erotic minds. When a man is focused only on his natural self without any spiritual balance, or when he has a twisted notion of what it means to be masculine, the natural balance of a sexual relationship is lost, and things can start to spin out of kilter. But it doesn't have to be this way!

Women have a part to play as well; they need to learn, as Anaïs Nin wrote, to "expose the purely macho type, his false masculinity, physical force, dexterity in games, arrogance, but more dangerous still, his lack of sensitivity." Reject the hero of Last Tango in Paris, *"the sadist, the man who humiliates woman, whose show of power is a facade." False heroes of masculinity need to be rejected, "the stance of a Hemingway or a Mailer in writing, the false* strength." No longer should women "be subjected to this display of power" that doesn't protect them.[5] Women need men who will connect not only with them emotionally—with kindness and love—but also with themselves.

This doesn't mean a man should abandon the impulsive, linear, physical side of his nature for the more sensitive side. This would be a mistake, because it too would produce an imbalance. Instead, he needs to recognize his unique masculinity, retain it, but sanctify it with love and balance it with his deeper self—the true wild man who is powerful in his linear masculinity, yet not savage or sadistic. This is the man who personifies healthy masculine sexuality—he is unafraid to connect with a complete woman in all her power and gentleness, but he refuses to oppress or abuse her. He respects and adores her. She is his romantic partner, his erotic other, his soul mate.

CHAPTER 17

Loss of Feminine Love

I shall make a new song
before the wind blows and it freezes and rains.
My lady (ma dona) is trying and testing me,
to find out how much I love her.
Well, no matter what quarrel she makes,
she will not loose me from her bond.
Rather I become her servant, surrender to her,
so she can write my name in her contract.

WILLIAM IX, DUKE OF AQUITAINE

Women today take great pride in being sexual equals with men, and in many ways they should feel this way. For too long in history, they'd been treated as inferiors. By the mid-twentieth century, they'd had enough, and they brought about change. This freedom has been wonderful. But it has left many women depleted, depressed, and desperate for something more. Equality hasn't given them what they want. That's because equality isn't what women really wanted—they should have aimed higher.

Once upon a time women were considered the emotional, sexual, and spiritual superiors to men, but now they have inadvertently knocked themselves off their own pedestal. This has been detrimental, not only to women, but to men. We're now out of balance, with the feminine fading from the relationship. Women need to find their sexual equilibrium, and men need to treat women as the prize they truly are. As women have begun to take on male traits in the bedroom, the feminine has been nearly lost and the sexual experience has been masculinized. The emotional and sensual connection that is so essential to our deepest sexual needs has been broken.

With this masculinization of sex, women have too often forgotten their feminine sensitivities and how they naturally feel the rhythms of life around them. Too many women, especially in America, have lost their sensuality. They've become desensitized and dulled by appropriating masculine rhythms, losing the vibrancy, sensuality, and power they—and men—so desperately need.

One of the sad results of this masculinization is men become the driving force of sex. This leads us to believe that men are more interested in sex than women are. But this simply isn't the case. It appears this way because feminine sexual power won't be present unless a man draws it out. It's the wild masculine that reaches under the outward layers of the woman's dual nature and pulls the wild feminine up from the depths where sensual fires burn, enveloping him in their heat.

But this isn't happening because it's all so easy. Women are on the surface with men, sex is shallow, desensitized. There's no feeling the sensations of a woman's circular sexuality. There's just a man's linear sexual experience. The orgasm is accomplished and they're done. Women remain closed off because their true passions are not ignited. The richness of their sexuality fades, their heat lies dormant, their fires turn to cold. This leads to disinterest and the general impression that women just aren't into sex as much as men. This has now become a cultural norm with sayings like "Women need a reason to have sex, men just need a place" and "Marriage is the price men pay for sex, and sex is the price women pay for marriage."

This, however, is far from the truth. In the past and in other cultures, the feminine presence was seen as more passionate than the masculine. Men were enraptured by a woman's powerful sexuality and intimidated by it. They had to earn the right to even stand in its presence. Husbands had to work hard to satisfy their wives so they wouldn't stray. A man's own sexuality was stimulated and invigorated by the power of the woman, creating tension and fueling his erotic needs.

One of the most illustrative images of the power of female sexuality and how it fuels masculine erotic love is the Hindu myth of Rati, the goddess of passion, lust, and sexual pleasure. As the only companion worthy of the great Kama, the male god of love and desire, her feminine power is not childbearing or childrearing. She has nothing to do with wifely duties. Rati is pure passion and pleasure, set apart to satisfy Kama. She ignites his desires and inflames his love. Her sensuality gives him life and enables him to spread love to others. Everything about Rati is sensual and feminine, and it is this feminine sexuality that arouses the erotic masculinity in Kama, just as his desire arouses her own erotic needs. They are a circle, not a line. He is drawn into her by the power of her sensuality.

The Hindu texts focus on this sensuality through descriptions of Rati's body. All five senses are touched on: "see her feet dyed red with henna like a bride, hear the jangling of her ankle bells . . . , feel the softness of her hair, smell the fragrance of her breath, and almost taste her presence as it might fill a room like the light of a full moon."[1] Kama, her male counterpart, can't resist as all of his senses are inflamed by her unbridled sexuality. A woman's sensuality is powerful when it is on full display, and men become weak in its presence.

This image of the sexual power of a woman is common throughout many cultures, but it is one we have lost, particularly in America where androgyny has robbed both men and women of passionate connectedness. The masculine erotic nature needs the power of the feminine; otherwise his heart, his mind, and all his senses are disconnected from sex. He's left with only his masculine impulses, linear, unbalanced, and uncivilized.

When women no longer embrace this powerful sensuality and, instead, act like men, the experience is colder. This is what happened when the equalizing of the sexes morphed into encouragement to mirror men. Women were told to have sex like men—physically oriented, emotionally disconnected, moving from one partner to another in the quest to find someone new. The orgasm, not intimacy, became the goal for many. They lost their feminine balance.

Many men have been led to believe that this new availability of sex is a great thing. But it has also incentivized behavior that is both indecorous—men treating women like trophies—and not conducive to happiness in male sexuality. It is now possible for men to sleep with several women one after another without emotional commitment. When women become pregnant, even though it takes two to tango, there is less expectation of male responsibility, leading to an unequal burden of responsibility on women. Modern sexual expectations encourage men to avoid the responsibilities and risks of marriage while still getting all the sex they can.

As fun as this might sound to some, it has led to deep dissatisfaction for both women and men. Women have been downgraded from their honored place as men's sexual counterparts and cherished companions. As a result, men are encouraged to cast women aside after using them, instead of adoring them. Many men have become coarsened by the consumerist approach to sexual partnership. The language in which many men discuss their romantic interests has also devolved, leaving them discontent, but unable to express or recognize why, because although their real erotic desires aren't being met, they have no language in which to express this.

As counterintuitive as it might sound, men need women to embrace the power of their femininity and to willingly exercise that power in their relationships. Men should have to earn a woman's trust, attention, and intimacy. This has an ennobling effect, because it encourages men to approach women as people rather than as objects of sexual gratification. Once a man has earned a woman's trust and intimacy, he is elevated above all other men in that woman's eyes and he is motivated to retain that honored place by keeping her satisfied and being the kind, loving, respectful man he should be.

RABBI SHMULEY

Throughout history and in many cultures, women have been considered the dominant civilizing force in society. They commit fewer crimes, they care for their children when men abandon them, they attend church and synagogue more than men do, they do more acts of service and are more community minded, and they bring cooperation where men focus on competition. Women, according to the Talmud, are "wiser than men," which is why in the Jewish religion the feminine day of the Sabbath is the most holy day. This emphasis on the valued nature of the feminine is also found in the term for the omnipresence of God: the "shechina," the feminine divine presence.

Women bring balance in a relationship by forcing men to face their emotional needs instead of focusing only on their physical sexual appetites. But as the difference between the sexes is eroded, women have fewer incentives to exercise this role. As a result, men have no incentive to focus on their deep needs. Instead they focus on their immediate sexual urges, and the cycle continues, driving the wedge between the sexes deeper and deeper. Many don't even realize their real desire is not for sex but to be needed by a woman and to find rest in her feminine embrace.

What our society needs, especially in America, is to learn from the courtly ideals of the past. Granted, even at their height in the twelfth century, these were not fully incorporated into the culture, but they were socially significant nonetheless. Courtly love was an ideal developed in France by Eleanor of Aquitaine and her daughter Marie, the Countess of Champagne, to bring civility, kindness, and mutual respect to the court.

Europe was emerging from the coarseness and brutality of the Dark Ages when women were treated as a man's property, and these influential, revolutionary women wanted change. They wanted to live in a more refined age. Masculine energies were dominant and unmoored from the civilizing influence of the feminine. Art and poetry during that time were filled with images of war, conflict, and male domination. To free women from their inferior role and unleash the gentle effects of femininity on society, Eleanor cultivated the arts and opened her court to the romantic poetry of the troubadours in which women were treated as goddesses.

It's interesting that in reaction to a brutal, oppressive period for women, Eleanor didn't champion equality for women, but their superiority. This, of course, might be because of her aristocratic status, but we think it had more to do with her understanding that women are more naturally refined when it comes to courtesy and kindness; they are gentler by nature and should be honored as such. Eleanor and the poets of courtly love wanted to bring feminine balance to society through romance and love. Of course, this exultation of women, particularly in marriage, was only an ideal and difficult to put into practice because marriages at the time were arranged and based, not on love, but family interests. Yet, these purveyors of romance knew the message of courtly love would have a leavening effect, at least on the upper echelons of society.

Courtly love was radical because it was based on European feudalism in which the knight was beholden to his lord, owing him fealty, devotion, and obedience. By this model, the man was obliged to the woman. She would be his master, and he would be her servant. Of course, only a great woman would deserve such dedication. Cruel, selfish, ignoble women would not be worthy of a man's pursuits—only one who would elevate him to be better, to be greater in every way, to fight for her and find gratification in his efforts to win her. He would pursue such a woman, night and day, to serve her. His heart would be enlarged by his quest. She was his golden chalice, his chosen one, his Isolde, his Guinevere. His desire for

her would overwhelm him to the point that he could not live without her.
He longed, as men still do today, even if they don't admit it, for her attention and her love. When he didn't get it, he was devastated.

The poetry of one of the most famous troubadours of the age, Arnaut
Daniel, describes this perfectly:

> I tell little of what's in my heart:
>
> fear makes me silent and scared;
>
> tongue hides but heart wants
>
> that on which, in pain, broods so:
>
> I languish, but I do not complain
>
> because so far
>
> as the sea embraces the earth
>
> there's none so kind,
>
> currently,
>
> as the chosen one
>
> for whom I long.[2]

The poets of courtly love understood that with great love, there is great
pain and at times suffering. Men took significant emotional risk to fall in
love with a noble and beautiful woman. But they believed it was worth it,
because she was worth it. "This love wounds my heart with a sweet taste,"
the troubadour Bernart de Ventadorn wrote, "so gently, I die of grief a
hundred times a day and a hundred times revive with joy."[3] The pain he
feels while waiting for his chosen one to return his affection was "worth
more than any pleasure"[4] because he knew, when she finally did yield to
his pursuit of her, the good result will be so much better "when this suffering is done."[5]

Today, this kind of romance is so rare as to appear almost quaint. Some
men are too afraid. They don't want to pursue a woman because they
don't want to get hurt. Opening their heart, after all, takes bravery, and

in the modern sexual marketplace, that kind of bravery is not rewarded. Other men have come to have their sensuality deadened or dulled by the easy availability of sex. Sexual consumerism has raised the risks for men of opening their hearts to women, but it has also drastically lowered the risks involved in seeking sex from women.

Many men have become stuck in this contradiction: they don't have to risk much of anything to get sex, and they don't have to convince women of their romantic interest in order to get it. In fact, the opposite is often true: some women give themselves over in every way to a man—even on the first date—to prove their worth to him. But it doesn't work, because there's no incentive to remain committed to her, no choosing, no special-ness, no loyalty. She doesn't need to inspire him, she needs only to sleep with him. She has offered him nothing to make him better, and he manages to go through the motions of romantic attraction without being enriched by it. She has sacrificed her feminine power by giving it away and letting it be consumed by uncontrolled masculine energy. In this way, neither men nor women stand to benefit from the civilizing effect of romantic courtship.

For the man, he is left empty because the truly erotic connection that satisfies his sensual soul is to have her reach out to him and say, "I need and want only you." It's this feminine sexuality—both in her powerful response and his emotional need—that creates the tension that sustains their love. He needs her and hungers for her, as Pablo Neruda wrote in his poem "I Crave Your Mouth, Your Voice, Your Hair."[6]

This is what a man wants. He wants feminine love, to capture it and consume it, to be surrounded by it as he is encircled by a woman's body when they make love. Instead, today we have the masculinization of love and women's feminine influence weakened in relationships. Life was much more romantic when women were more empowered—and relationships were a lot more passionate.

In a way, we're right back in the dark ages with a coarse, hedonistic sexuality and an ideal of masculinity that is about male sexual dominance rather than strength and commitment in love. To rediscover the lost art of intimacy, we need to do something radical, just as Eleanor of Aquitaine did. We need to become activists for the cause of passionate connectedness: to bring back kindness, courtesy, and respect in our relationships; to put one another first; to pursue and be pursued; to be brave in the face of possible rejection; to be vulnerable. We need—all of us desperately need—a revival of the feminine.

CHAPTER 18

Cheating: It's Not All About Sex

*We aren't who we want to be. We are what society demands. We
are what our parents choose. We don't want to disappoint anyone;
we have a great need to be loved. So we smother the best in us.*

PAULO COELHO

Pamela

*Early in my career, when I was beginning to find success as a model, my
mother joked that my success would doom me to a life of loneliness. Being
able to earn my place in the world would give me independence, my mother
predicted, and this would emasculate any man I met. "Never make more
money than your man," she told me one evening, with a glint in her eye.
"Or, if you do . . . LIE!"*

It may have been a joke, but there is some truth to it too. From the
day they are born, men are told they must be strong, independent, and
aggressive. In their relationships with women, they are encouraged to be
the protector, the provider, and the householder. This is still the case,
despite the fact that there is more equality between the sexes now. Men
are made to feel as if failing to meet this ideal is failing to be a man.

Society convinces them that if they do not feel the burden of responsibility on their shoulders, there is something wrong with them. In a real sense, our society sets men up to be unhappy in the twenty-first century because it gives them expectations of the relations between the sexes that cannot always satisfy their need to be the breadwinner.

This doesn't mean that women should return to the condition of subordination to men in marriage. Before female emancipation, women were passed from father to husband as property. Women had no financial independence from men and had no agency of their own. This was an awful state of affairs. The equality of the sexes was an important and necessary development, which reformed these institutions and saw women achieve freedom from oppressive subordination to men.

Women should obviously not be financially enslaved by their husbands. Doing so not only subverts female potential and talent but also produces conditions whereby women can be exploited or manipulated. It creates a real and harmful power difference between men and women.

Pamela

I understand this situation very well—I have had relationships in the past when my partner encouraged me to depend on him financially, but he then tried to use that dependency to manipulate me. Financial independence for women is a good thing. Women should have their own careers, operate autonomously in the world, and in real terms be the equals of their partners. This fosters mutual respect in a marriage, a cooperative ethos, and a sense of equality that is to be desired in a relationship.

But at the same time, women must be sensitive to the emotional and psychological needs of their partner. They must understand that the need to feel strong can be a weakness in men. And in a relationship, men and women support each other and compensate for each other's weaknesses. A woman must understand that—even if he understands and respects her need for real equality in a relationship—he has still been conditioned by a society that places a heavy emphasis on the stereotype of the male protector, the male provider. There will be times when he needs—for his own sense of worth—to feel as if he is providing for his woman, protecting her and sustaining her: being the man of the house. And in those times, perhaps the woman may not want to wound his self-esteem by denying him this experience.

This is not submission to patriarchal tradition—it is better to understand it as having the delicacy and the sensitivity to live harmoniously in a relationship with a man. Female independence also means a woman having the freedom and the autonomy and common sense not to torment her man or emasculate him by rubbing his face in her success or acting as if she doesn't really need him. It is a given in any true marriage that men and women need each other. And notwithstanding how nice it is to be independent and free, it is also nice sometimes to be protected and provided for—to feel the comfort and security of a strong and competent person taking care of things.

Regardless of the push and pull of married life—shared home, shared responsibilities, and shared finances—it is in a couple's erotic life that this lesson must most be understood, because it is there that our most basic emotional needs become more obvious. Sexually satisfying our partners requires that we understand those needs. And for many men, this means the need—at least some of the time—to take control, to lead. It is the need for his strength and physicality and passion to play a role in sex.

This doesn't mean a woman should always be submissive or sycophantic, always genuflecting to her man or appeasing his vanity or emotional neediness. It means recognizing those needs as a factor in the psychology of a relationship. It means addressing them—intelligently and sensitively. The depth and complexity of the female and male erotic minds should be something a couple tries to explore and understand together, so that they can experiment with it, even play and have fun with it, and, having come to a better understanding of it, grow closer together. As two people together, they can accept each other as they are and enrich their marriage and erotic life.

When this doesn't happen, affairs are often the result, and the most destructive force to relationships is infidelity. It sweeps away the unsuspecting like a storm, leveling everything in its path. Lives are torn apart, hearts are broken, and dreams are destroyed. We see this in the Book of Malachi, when God's people "cover the altar of the Lord with tears, with weeping and groaning" because he is no longer accepting their offerings with favor. They wonder why, and this is the Lord's response: "Because the Lord has been a witness between you and the wife of your youth, against whom you have dealt treacherously, though she is your companion and your wife by covenant."[1] Infidelity results not only in physical and relationship loss, but also in spiritual desolation.

Adultery is one of the great themes of human experience, illustrated not only in religious texts and the annals of history but in great works of literature. Tolstoy's *Anna Karenina*. Flaubert's *Madame Bovary*. Fitzgerald's *Tender Is the Night*. Percy's *Love in Ruins*. Charlotte Bronte's *Jane Eyre*—this last being full of mystery, passion, and romance, but with infidelity at its core. Sophisticated, wealthy, and married (albeit to a crazy woman), Mr. Rochester chooses a plain governess to fill his empty heart. So desperate is his need for a woman's love that he calls her "my rescuer." When she leaves him, this powerful man is reduced to sobs, throwing himself on the sofa and crying, "Oh, Jane! my hope, my love, my life."

Not every affair is as dramatic—or justifiable—as this one. But it does illustrate a point about men and adultery that bears repeating: Most men cheat, not for sex, but for emotional connection—to have someone meet the deep needs of their soul, allowing them to rest in feminine acceptance, appreciation, and love.

As we've seen, men are judged by their external actions—their successes, accomplishments, and abilities to provide, protect, and produce.

This creates a great deal of emotional stress for men. They don't express it the way women do, but they feel it. The need to always prove themselves can wear them down, and if they're not bolstered within themselves through faith and love, they will become broken. They will feel like failures, even if they're successful, rich, and living a life that most people would envy.

According to Aristotle, highly successful men are by nature melancholy and often inwardly broken in some way. They try to prove to themselves through external success that they have internal value. This is why they so desperately seek to be loved by the public. They need constant affirmation. Men like this are always teetering on the edge of obscurity. One slip, and they disappear. They base their value on the perceptions of others instead of finding it within themselves and discovering their self-worth in who they are, not merely what they do. This causes them to live in a constant state of insecurity. It's why they secretly question their value and why they turn to women to feel desirable and to find comfort in the midst of their inward pain.

When men don't feel like they're being validated in their relationships, they will often look for it from others. Most men who cheat aren't "bad" people, but they are broken inside. They're insecure and they need someone to affirm them and appreciate who they are. They often think they're getting this when a woman outside their marriage pays attention to them. They're drawn to the woman out of a deep need, and that emotional need is expressed through sex. Often, though, the "attention" he thinks he's getting isn't real. There isn't the emotional connection he's really wanting—or he doesn't realize himself that this is what he's actually looking for—and so he moves on to another woman. Men like this, addicted to the ephemeral rush of a false connection, are at risk of becoming womanizers, hoping that a long line of women will somehow make them feel complete and heal their brokenness.

Men want to feel powerful and important. They want to feel like a winner and on top of the world. Low self-esteem and the desire to feel desired and appreciated often push them to find validation outside of their marriages. Adultery rarely happens in a vacuum. Very often infidelity exposes cracks that were already in the relationship or a man who feels expendable and who seeks to feel essential. This is not the fault of his wife, and the cheating spouse must take responsibility for his actions. But whether the neglect is real or imagined, the worst remedy is finding validation outside of the marriage. You don't fix what's broken about you by adding dysfunction and complications. You fix it by fixing your relationship. The emotional wounds of being a man in today's world need the healing powers of the feminine.

Men who are suffering need the attention of a woman to soothe their broken egos. When a woman cares for a man, makes herself available to him, and tells him how wonderful he is, it becomes a salve, healing his soul. When this is happening within a marriage—in a myriad of different ways—men are satisfied and less likely to stray. When they're looking for this from other women, it can become addictive as they experience a false intimacy that doesn't last and is ultimately unfulfilling. A sense of emptiness takes hold, usually before they even get out of bed and dress to return home.

Sometimes this need for intimacy and validation doesn't involve sex. Most affairs by husbands aren't physical at all. They're over the phone or online, and they're never consummated. Men talk to one woman after another online, in chat rooms, or via texting to get the attention they crave. But it's never enough. They always need more and keep looking, typing away at the computer keys in search of connection.

As long as we continue to think men cheat for sex, we will never heal our relationships. We will miss the root problem. We won't learn to love. We won't discover answers to our often unspoken questions. "Life offers us thousands of opportunities for learning," Paulo Coelho writes in *Adultery*. We just need to be open to learn and change. "Every man and every woman, in every day of our lives, always has a good opportunity to sur-render to love. Life is not a long vacation but a learning process. And the most important lesson is learning to love. Loving better and better."[2]

Before we can learn to love, we need to understand our needs, phys-ically and emotionally. Men have deep emotional needs, and many are experiencing hidden brokenness because they have never had those needs met. Gary Neuman, a fellow rabbi and friend of Rabbi Shmuley, has done extensive research into why men cheat. "[F]or all of their sexual prowess, needs, and desires, the majority of men are not on the lookout for a new fantastic sex voyage with another woman," he writes in *The Truth about Cheating*. "They are looking for emotional connection."[3]

In a survey of men who had cheated on their wives, Neuman found that the main drivers of their infidelity were emotional dissatisfaction (48 per-cent) and equal emotional and sexual dissatisfaction (32 percent):[4]

> *Among all of the possible causes of emotional dissatisfaction the most common answer was, "I felt underappreciated by my wife. She was not sufficiently thoughtful and car-ing toward me." This response made up 37 percent of the emotional problems for these men. Consider also that "I felt emotionally disconnected from my wife" represented 17 percent of the problems they felt. Together, these two answers that clearly relate to their wives' appreciation, thoughtfulness, and emotional connection represent 54 percent of the emotional dissatisfaction that cheating men believed helped lead them into the arms of another woman. The feeling of under-appreciation and lack of thoughtfulness far outweighed any other choice on the list.*[5]

To put it simply, "[m]en need to hear how wonderful they are and to be appreciated for what they do right," Neuman writes. "They may not talk emotionally, may not say things like, 'When you speak that way it makes me feel . . .' but make no mistake, they are emotional beings who are look-ing for warmth, kindness, and appreciation."[6]

Being underappreciated is not an excuse to cheat in marriage. None of us has a justification for immoral action, and each of us has to be accountable for our actions. If you feel underappreciated in your marriage, it's either because it's real, in which you case you have to repair it, or it's because it's a fantasy in your mind, in which case you have to get over it. Either way, adultery is never a solution. Acknowledging and addressing genuine male and female emotional needs in a relationship is key.

All of this mirrors the impossible expectations placed on men and women in our society. Today's women are told throughout their childhood that they can have it all and be whatever they want to be—and we encourage women to both pursue their dreams and live an authentic life. But too many women are nowadays stuck between a rock and a hard place—they believe they must have a great career and be a great wife and mother too. Sometimes these are irreconcilable and unrealistic expectations, given the pressures of a modern life. There just isn't time to do all of this. The same can be said about men. In these modern times, there are more expectations on men as well. They, too, are facing demands like never before—to be perfect in the home and in the workplace.[7]

When your abilities and values are judged by what you do and accomplish, these added expectations only add to the burden men have. When they feel like they've failed because they receive no validation, they're broken inside. They need encouragement and appreciation too, and they shouldn't be ashamed to express that need. Sadly, our culture shames them into silence because they're supposed to be the emotionally self-sufficient ones in the relationship. This simply isn't the case. "As far forward as society has moved in not placing people into categories just because of gender," Neuman writes, "men are still thought of as the ones primarily responsible for protecting and providing financially for the family. Appreciation for their work in this area is often missed by wives."[8]

One extreme solution that might be proposed is for more men to simply abandon the outmoded, traditional idea of the male provider, and let the wife be the breadwinner. Without all the added pressure of competition and needing to provide, men will be happier, right? Actually, not always. A study published in the *American Sociological Review* found that men who were "100% economically dependent on their spouses were most at risk for cheating, three times more at risk than women married to male bread-winners."[9] And this is unsurprising, because why should men find it easier to be 100 percent economically dependent on their spouses than women did in the past? There remains in our culture a strong pressure on men to validate themselves and affirm their masculinity by providing for their families. If a man feels emasculated, weak, unappreciated, or insignificant, he will often search for meaning and validation elsewhere.

This, however, does not ever justify an affair. When a man breaks his vows and finds solace and sex in another woman, he is solely to blame for this choice. There are reasons he is tempted to cheat—and that's the point we're making—but his choice to cheat instead of facing his real issues is *his* fault, not his partner's. He might not be having his emotional and/or sexual needs met, but that doesn't give him license to commit adultery, just as it doesn't give a woman the right to have an affair if her husband doesn't desire her as he should. We are not driven by our emotional impulses without any sense of responsibility. We might be suffering and deprived within a relationship, but this doesn't legitimize hurting the one we love to get our needs met from another.

We must also recognize that there are some men (Neuman found it to be about 12 percent) who cheat just to cheat, and women who are caught in this twisted web of pure selfishness need compassion and help to deal with a difficult circumstance. But that still leaves 88 percent of men who might not have cheated if their self-esteem had not been so low.[10] Men are emotional creatures and require passionate connectedness with their partners.

For these men, it's not just about sex. If all they wanted was sex, they'd stay with their wives. They don't even want interesting or better sex—often men who cheat say sex with the mistress isn't that great. It's emotional. They need the healing attentions of their partner, not just once in a while, but often. This appreciation, for men, is very much connected with sex, but sex is not the central need. In the erotic life of a married couple, sex is important, but it is also the conduit for the emotional connection that supports and sustains them. Emotional appreciation is shown through meaningful, passionate sex within a relationship. Showing consideration and sensitivity in all areas of a marriage is crucial, but one of the best ways a woman can show her appreciation is not only with her words, but with her actions—by making love to her man. The touch a man needs is that of the woman he loves in the context of kindness and appreciation. This will arouse his erotic mind. It will stimulate his body and his heart. It will form a passionate connection that is essential to a healthy relationship.

Women, through no fault of their own, don't always know a man's deepest needs because men often struggle to reveal them. Women aren't mind readers, and men don't always open up. It's up to men to be emotionally available and tell their wives what they need—and that takes some self-reflection and vulnerability. The fear of failure is often lingering in the back of their minds, haunting them. They need to be honest with their partners about this or they won't find the healing they need.

"Men who learn to talk to their wives about their deepest fears slowly become immune to an affair," Rabbi Shmuley wrote in an article titled "Why Men Cheat and How They Can Be Stopped." "Infidelity, it turns out, often provides a starting point for couples to address the void in their relationship which usually consists of the lack of truly intimate communication about life's anxieties and apprehensions. A man's deepest fear is of failure. And the person he most masks this from is his own wife because she is the person whose opinion matters most. I know husbands who have been laid off from their jobs in this recession who still put on a suit every day and leave the house so that their wives never find out. So called 'successful' men harbor the same fears. And rather than destructively address the fear by becoming a stud to other women, he can purge from himself a dependency on strangers by learning to confide fully in his wife."[11]

Pamela

The message here is really rather simple—it's about kindness. It's about love—both giving in equal measure. When we don't have it, we're hurting and lonely. Cheating, for some, is like a gasp of air when you're drowning. Men feel like they're drowning under the weight of expectations and failures. They feel as if they're worthless. When they're not needed, they can't breathe. Women feel this way when they're no longer desired. They feel hollow, as if they're a mere ghost walking the halls of their home.

Both can be freed from these turbulent waters with kindness—a sensual kindness that touches their bodies and souls. In this, they give each other what they need to be whole. As we've discovered, within a heterosexual relationship, a man desperately needs a woman, and a woman desperately needs a man—the masculine and the feminine, together, complete. Men have their unique differences and needs, as do women. We need to celebrate those differences instead of ignoring or ridiculing them. Failing to do so divides us, driving us out the door and into the arms of others or into isolated corners where we weep alone.

This doesn't need to be the fate of relationships, but change has to start from within, from realizing that our souls need to be fed and not just our bodies—or vice versa. We have sacrificed living vibrant, sensual, spiritually rich lives for the robotic existence of materialism, isolation, and disconnected sex. Too many people have forgotten how to *be* in love. They have forgotten the deep waters and raging fires that dwell within all of us. Men have forgotten how to ignite a woman's fire, and women have forgotten how to swim into the depths of a man's soul. When a man forgets how to love a woman and a woman forgets how to love a man, they will drift apart. As the one lets go, so will the other. "If suddenly you forget me, do not look for me, for I shall already have forgotten you," Neruda writes.[12]

Our hope in writing this book is to help couples remember how to love and never forget to taste its sweetness, to see its glow in each other's eyes, to feel its gentle touch against their skin, to smell its burning embers of passion, and to hear its power—and its comfort—in the tender whispers of "I love you." The next two parts will give practical advice on how to do just this by infusing relationships with curiosity, mystery, spiritual connection, and even a little naughtiness.

Part Five

PILLARS OF EROTICISM

CHAPTER 19

Unavailability

I have seen romanticism outlast the realistic. I have seen men forget the beautiful women they have possessed, forget the prostitutes, and remember the first woman they idolized, the woman they could never have. The woman who aroused them romantically holds them.

ANAÏS NIN

Venice, Italy. Henry James described her "an orange gem resting on a blue glass plate." Arthur Symons said she had the power to turn a realist into a romantic "by mere faithfulness to what he saw before him." This "white swan of cities," as Henry Wadsworth Longfellow called it, has inspired many an artist, poet, and lover. So taken with her magical beauty, Percy Bysshe Shelley tried to capture her essence in rhyme, the words pouring breathlessly from his pen:

> *Underneath day's azure eyes,*
> *Ocean's nursling, Venice, lies,—*
> *A peopled labyrinth of walls,*
> *Amphitrite's destined halls,*
> *Which her hoary sire now paves*

With his blue and beaming waves.

Lo! the sun upsprings behind,

Broad, red, radiant, half reclined

On the level quivering line

Of the waters crystalline;

And before that chasm of light,

As within a furnace bright,

Column, tower, and dome, and spire

Shine like obelisks of fire,

Pointing with inconstant motion

From the altar of dark ocean

To the sapphire-tinted skies;

As the flames of sacrifice

From the marble shrines did rise,

As to pierce the dome of gold

Where Apollo spoke of old.

Sun-girt city! thou hast been

Ocean's child, and then his queen.[1]

This is Venice. Her "flattering and suspect beauty"[2] inspires the arts and a sleepy eroticism that teases the soul and the imagination. Venice is one of the most beautiful and erotic cities in the world because she embodies the qualities that fuel desire—mystery, forbiddenness, and unavailability. Her streets are difficult to maneuver. It's easy to get lost in the city, among the water, the passageways, the bridges and lanes—you end up in places you never intended to go, creating a sense of anticipation and unavailability. It's the city of seduction. Everywhere you go there is hidden history, ancient stories whispering from her walls, echoes of days long past drifting on the breeze among her domes and towers, secrets floating on her waters, disappearing with the tide. When night descends, lights cast their glow softly across her face, creating an erotic allure filled with mystery.

Venice is illustrative of erotic unavailability—something we need in our relationships, something essential to rediscovering intimacy. We wonder why our sexual relationships are so stagnant. Why are we tempted by strangers? Why do we think monogamy is impossible and long-term relationships are doomed to fail? Because we've lost erotic desire, passionate connection, and sensuality. Our relationships have become dry and monotonous because we haven't kept the flames of desire alive.

One reason for this is we've become too familiar in our relationships. Long-term partners lose interest because they already know everything about each other. Predictable routines and too much availability will kill a marriage. When couples do the same things repeatedly, walk the same paths, eat at the same restaurants, repeat the same mundane conversations, have sex at the same time for ten or fifteen minutes, distance creeps into the relationship. They often don't even talk because they already know what the other is going to say. When they do talk, they finish each other's sentences.

It's an ever-present danger, dealing with the monotony of everyday life. The more routine everything becomes, the more two people run the risk of collapsing into one. There is of course a romantic way of speaking about marriage: "two hearts become one." But this is a figure of speech. In reality, you need to be two people together to get the most out of companionship. You can't forget the other person exists. To do so is almost to forget your own existence.

We know adultery is most often caused by lack of emotional connection, laziness, and neglect. When couples look at each other without interest because they're too familiar, the temptation to stray increases. What they need is to become less available to each other. Unavailability is frustrated desire, an erotic obstacle. It's when an impediment stands between you and the object of your desire. To rediscover intimacy and passion, we have to learn to embrace hunger rather than rushing to satiate every desire. This constant instant gratification inevitably leads to boredom.

Steve Jobs of Apple understood this concept well and applied it to business. One of the first things he did was make his products hard to get. If you didn't arrive at the store early in the morning to buy the newest iPhone, you wouldn't get one. You'd have to wait for the next shipment. Hundreds of people would stand in line for hours just to get an iPhone. One summer in New York, Apple had to deliver bottled water to keep customers from getting overheated and fainting. That's how desperate people were to have an iPhone. They were like lovers, aching to see the object of their desire, a line of Romeos at Juliet's balcony. It was just a phone, but it had erotic appeal, which Jobs ingeniously superimposed on a material object, ensuring devoted customers.

Jobs grasped something important about human nature and desire: If you make something hard to get, people will want it more. Love and friendship are about familiarity and availability, but desire and passion are about unavailability. After all, is it even possible to want something, to lust after it, to desire it, if you already have it? The first principle of desire is to long for something you can't have because once you have it, that fire will grow cold—and quickly. To keep the flames of passion alive, there has to be some measure of unavailability injected into the relationship.

Unavailability is one of the elements that makes the *Song of Solomon* so erotic. Never are the lovers described as satiating their hunger for each other. They are always just missing that glorious moment of consummation. They live in a state of frustrated desire:

> *All night long on my bed*
> *I looked for the one my heart loves;*
> *I looked for him but did not find him.*
> *I will get up now and go about the city,*
> *through its streets and squares;*
> *I will search for the one my heart loves.*
> *So I looked for him but did not find him.*

The watchmen found me

as they made their rounds in the city.

"Have you seen the one my heart loves?"[3]

Erotic desire is awakened through obstacles and absence. It's only soothed through satiation and fulfillment. Desire is unfulfilled longing that thrives in separation, not familiarity.

Everyone has at some point experienced unavailability—being away from your lover for a week or two and then coming back to him or her. And we know that feeling when we return, the eagerness to see them again, maybe even a tiny bit of doubt: "Did he miss me as much as I missed him?" That feeling when you can finally be together and intimate again is different from routine togetherness. The absence, the unavailability, has added something. The slight estrangement introduces that little bit of added electricity into our caress, that little bit more fire into our kiss. And the secret to keeping a relationship burning is learning how to cultivate this feeling, how to maintain it, so that we feel it even when we haven't been apart.

All the great romances have this relationship between unavailability and desire woven into them. Catherine and Heathcliff in *Wuthering Heights*. Scarlett's longing for Ashley Wilkes in *Gone with the Wind*. Elizabeth and Mr. Darcy's unlikely courtship in *Pride and Prejudice*. The tragedy of forbidden love in *Romeo and Juliet*. One of the greatest examples of passion and unavailability is James Getz's obsession with the unattainable Daisy in *The Great Gatsby*.

The son of struggling farmers, Getz fell in love with a girl out of his league, and he changed his life and name to become a man worthy of her. He spent years thinking of her, his imagination enlarged and his passion swelling. His thoughts dwelt on her—an image, a myth, forming in his mind. He magnified her, making much more of her than she really was. He threw himself into "a creative passion," and nothing would change his mind about her: "no amount of fire or freshness can challenge what a man will store up in his ghostly heart."[4]

This anticipation, the distance between them, even their profound differences—all heightened his desire. So intense was this feeling, so great his flights of ecstasy at the mere thought of her, that he didn't want to be brought down to earth, even as he stood on the cusp of his dreams becoming a reality:

> His heart beat faster and faster as Daisy's white face came up to his own. He knew that when he kissed this girl, and forever wed his unutterable visions to her perishable breath, his mind would never romp again like the mind of God. So he waited, listening for a moment longer to the tuning-fork that had been struck upon a star. Then he kissed her. At his lips' touch she blossomed for him like a flower and the incarnation was complete.[5]

Unavailability forces us to expend mental energy. If there's no mental energy, there's no eroticism. Gatsby is an extreme example—we don't want so much distance that we fall in love with an illusion. But we do want our minds to be engaged, to seek knowledge of the other person, to anticipate what they're like, the sound of their voice, the touch of their skin, the smell of their hair, the taste of their lips.

The mind, not the body, is the source of pleasure and erotic longing. It is the primary sexual organ. If we have instant gratification and constant availability, our minds are disengaged. There's no real participating. It's like stuffing ourselves with potato chips, never really tasting them. When the mind is not given the opportunity to participate in longing, lust, and desire, we have relegated it to irrelevance. It's not participating. Once we've done that, we're casting aside the most important sensual organ. The brain processes all the senses. When something is instantly available, it's cut out of the process.

The essence of erotic longing is hunger. If you satiate the appetite immediately, you've removed hunger and pleasure. There's no involvement of the mind, no contemplation, no absorption of sensuality. You're reduced to a mere physical procedure—copulation. When you circumvent the mind, you're ignoring the single most important erogenous zone. You've diminished everything. There can be no sensuality. Sex still works but it's entirely physical, automatic. Human beings are unique because of the mind's participation. As Pamela says, brains are sexy! Without the involvement of the intellect, sex is just a compulsive, mechanical activity. Unavailability makes sex profoundly human as the mind plays a central role; it's a magnifier and force multiplier. It heightens the object of your desire.

Think about it. When you've been away on a trip and you come home, you're much more interested in your partner, especially if you've been spending time flirting on the phone or sending each other playful texts. Being forced to contain your desire for days instead of instantly satisfying it as you would have if you were home increases the intensity of that need. Your mind becomes engaged. You're thinking about it, imagining the curves of her body or the strength of his kiss. Sensuality is magnified, heating up your passion until it's painful. You hurt and ache for your lover because you can't have them, and when you do, it's so much better and the release much more satisfying.

We talk about the heart as the seat of the emotions, but it is only the pump that fuels the other organs. The real seat of emotions is the brain. Our minds make emotional and sensual connections. When we slow down and let the mind wander, contemplate, imagine, and create, passion grows and love expands. Eroticism infuses thought into the sexual experience. It brings together the material and spiritual, the finite and infinite. When the mind is involved, passion never fades, because the mind is the seat of desire and it's always active with imagination. It's the principal sex organ. The more the mind is engaged in sex, the more intensely erotic it becomes. This is why intelligence can be so sexy.

This is why men try to seduce women with poetry and intelligent conversation when they first meet—the brain is the seat of sexuality. An intellectually engaging man, a man who understands the world and can speak about it with confidence—these can be outrageously sexy characteristics. The same is true of women. It is a tremendous cliché that men only care about the physical. It's much more interesting for both parties if there is a mental spark, a spiritual connection, an understanding. The chemistry of a relationship, the erotic, lives in our conversation as much as it does in our physicality.

A man who engages a woman's mind, not just her body, is drawing her into his world, allowing her to get to know him at a deeper level, and setting her imagination on fire. The same is true for a woman when she talks with a man. Meeting someone who is knowledgeable is arousing because you want them to know you too, to peel back your layers and expose the essence of who you are.

People in long-term relationships often lose this spark because, in the push and pull of daily life, they let their minds go numb and their intellectual connection go to pasture. Their brains have become lazy, and the passion has withered. Instead of reading books before they go to bed, they watch television or read tabloids. Instead of having an interesting conversation at dinner or afterward as they sit on the porch with one another, they talk about work schedules, health issues, or what the neighbors are doing. Perhaps they don't even have time to speak at all. They don't realize that taking the time to engage each other with meaningful conversation is the early stage of foreplay. When two people are mentally engaged, they discover new things together, explore the world together, get to know each other over and over again, and they see each other in a new light.

They say "familiarity breeds contempt." We wouldn't go that far. But it's actually worse in some ways. At least contempt is an emotion! Familiarity doesn't breed contempt. It breeds indifference. That's the worst thing ever, to become sexually indifferent to your partner, even while you love them. Instead we have to learn to make our familiarity mean something. It should be *knowledge* of each other, an ability to love each other more expertly, not a blanket to smother everything exciting and sexy about our lives.

When we're too familiar or repeating the same habits over and over again, we get restless. It can happen with the most interesting man in the world or the most beautiful and fascinating woman. Even great works of genius can become boring if we're too familiar with them or if they're too available.

RABBI SHMULEY

When I was traveling in Europe, I went to the Palazzo Pitti, the Palace of the Medici, in Florence, Italy. In one of the rooms, there were several works by the great artist Raphael. I was mesmerized by them because I rarely have the opportunity to see such genius. Seeing even one can be a once-in-a-lifetime treat. But seeing so many in a room together lessened the impact. I noticed how so many people walked past them, interested, yes, but not as seriously appreciative or engaged. Faced with so many masterpieces by the same artist all in one room dampened the sense of awe, unavailability, and mystery.

The same was true at the Medici Chapel with the sculptures of Michelangelo. There were about four all in one small chapel, and people were no longer in awe of them. It was nothing like in America where Michelangelo's works are rarely shown. In 1964, his masterpiece *Pieta* was moved from the Vatican and brought to New York where it was put on display at the World's Fair. Thousands flocked to see it. Americans were captivated by it because they had never seen an original Michelangelo sculpture. It was rare, and the rarity of it, the unavailability of it, inspired them and excited them. It was akin to an erotic experience of rapture and longing.

When something is different from the norm, unavailable, and distant, there is a strong sense of otherness about it. We're drawn to that which is dissimilar, to people who are different from us, who stimulate our minds and invite us in to know something new. The entire attraction of sex is that it is with someone else. The other person adds something that we cannot add ourselves. There is no such thing as intimacy with yourself. It's the communication between two centers of awareness that makes sex electric. And it's all down to there being a "someone who is not me," who we do not fully understand. That's why it's important not to become so set in our ways that we forget it is another person we are with.

When something is easily available to us, we get to know it—at least the surface of it—and we integrate it into ourselves quickly. It moves at lightning speed from otherness to sameness. Sameness is boring because it doesn't inspire the imagination or give us energy to seek deeper knowledge. Unavailability does that for us as we look to connect with something outside our reach. It's not just that people want what they don't have. It's so much more than that. Unavailability maintains a sense of otherness.

But how can unavailability be maintained in a long-term relationship, with someone you eat with every day and sleep with every night, a body whose nakedness you see on a daily basis? Isn't sameness inevitable? It doesn't have to be. People are deep and complex (something we'll explore in the following chapters). Our sexual differences alone are rooted in otherness. The masculine and the feminine complement each other, helping to introduce this elusive sense of difference, staving off weariness and boredom. There is a profound dimension of otherness in a woman. She is mysterious and can't be fully realized. Men too! Even our anatomies are profoundly different—mysteries to be explored. A woman's inner sexuality has hidden erotic depths, and a man can spend a lifetime exploring this natural unavailability with one woman. When the mind is fully engaged and the correct level of unavailability is successfully maintained between a man and a woman, passion is sustained over time. There's always something new and exciting to learn from the one you're with—if you take the time to develop it and savor it in one another.

Unfortunately, too often we look for passion in the wrong places because we've become too familiar and we live only on the surface with each other, focusing mostly on the physical. We long to feel that spark of passion again, and many people look for it in new lovers. But this is a shallow and physically oriented tendency; it doesn't feed the need for erotic experience. When we move constantly from one partner to another, we don't develop the mental energies and the emotional depth that is necessary to sustain a genuinely erotic connection. Instead of looking outward, we need to look inward, within ourselves and our relationships. Unavailability is a big part of that.

Emotional separation awakens curiosity and longing between two people because what we want is emotional connection. Think about how passionate sex is after an argument. Arguments are often an instinctual renewal of our sexual connection. In many healthy relationships, especially between two powerful personalities, respectful but passionate disagreements are just part of the relationship. They are part of the cycle, part of how things are worked out, like seasons: growth and renewal.

When a couple argues, the emotional distance caused by the disagreement suddenly makes you seem new to each other once the argument is over. You want to reconnect with this person who was separated from you. This obviously doesn't mean that couples should fight more, but it does teach us a lesson—that separation can be erotic. A sense of forbiddenness is created when you can't have the person you want. When you're apart and then you come together, it makes your bodies feel novel. Your partner seems more interesting, and you learn new things about them when they're put outside of the context of everyday life.

Studies show that the main reason women cheat is neglect. Interestingly enough, the minute a husband discovers his wife is someone else's mistress, she often stops being boring to him. She's no longer perceived as a complacent wife who doesn't like sex. Suddenly he sees her once more as a sexual being. His response? He wants to have sex with her. It's not just for reestablishing control over her or reclaiming the sexual gifts of her body. If he wanted that, he'd lock her in the house. It's because he is now excited by her. She's something new and, in a way, unavailable.

To be sure, people should not cheat or swing to help their marriages. Adultery is a catastrophe for relationships, and open marriages are extremely volatile arrangements that have a very high probability of wreaking havoc on intimacy and trust. They're unhealthy and destructive. The real solution is to have the affair *with your partner*. Cheat with each other. The goal for a husband is to see his wife as powerfully sexual creature, a potential mistress, not simply a wife. Likewise, wives need to strive to see their husbands as admirers and lovers who want to sweep them away into fantasy.

Pamela

I was privileged to have been raised by colorful women. One of them was my great aunt, Auntie Vie. She was an immortal character in my life, a joyful person, but she had a tragic story to tell. Not everyone is lucky enough to meet the love of their life, but Vie met hers early, and their marriage was passionate and intense. It was always roses and wine with him, even though he drove her crazy at times. Tragically, having found her true love, she lost him too. He was a logger, and one day he was killed in a terrible accident at work. Although Vie always approached life with such verve, you could tell that losing her soul mate had hurt her beyond words. You could still see it in her eyes when she spoke. You could hear the years of loss behind her words, the loneliness she had felt. She never married again. But she was not defined by her loss. She was a very bright, effervescent, vivacious person, always the most glamorous person in the room, always sporting a feather boa: a beautiful force of nature in my life. All of these traits stayed with her, merely tempered by her experiences. She earned her wisdom.

Vie always had advice for those around her. A few years ago, before she died, she published a book full of it, Pickles to Pearls. *I remember vividly one piece of advice she used to give to me.* "Marriage is a life sentence," *Vie said.* "No man can do it all. You need one for conversation, one for a lover, one for presents, one for wine." "Be the mistress," *she told me.* "Never be the wife to your husband. Then you don't have to deal with the drudgery, and you get much more presents!"

I still think of Vie's advice when I talk about the art of keeping a relationship fresh. There is something about Vie's playful realism that I find refreshing: One partner cannot be enough, but this is what is romantic about passionate commitment to each other. Being with someone doesn't mean a moralistic injunction against having meaningful, fun relationships with other people. And I don't believe every marriage should be saved if the cost is too high—people should not stay in a relationship that makes them miserable.

Instead, the knowledge that "one partner cannot be enough" is a challenge to us to find the many people in each of us, so that we will be adequate to each other. If marriage is to work, it must have a tolerance for the need for novelty in each of us, but in recognition of this, we must also strive to be many people for our partners: the constant companion, the passionate lover, the giver of gifts, the flirt, the person to talk to, the person to go on adventures with, the protector, the comrade, the friend, the person to argue with, the grounded one, and, yes, sometimes the critic. Being together is a constant striving down into the depths to find all of these different people within ourselves and discovering them in our partner. Some of the richest rewards in life are to be found in this kind of relationship. It is this secret, this knowledge that we are still potentially in competition with others for the attention of our partner that reminds us that they are a person with needs and desires, keeping us on our toes, holding our relationships in tension, and banishing drudgery from our lives together.

It's also very important in long-term relationships not to make sex commonplace or to allow it to lose its allure. This doesn't mean couples should play manipulative games with each other, denying each other for sadistic pleasure or turning sex on and off like a tap to control their partners. Healthy couples should be having regular sex to keep their relationship alive. But it is important to be conscious of the need for unavailability. This means they should approach their sex lives with a keen mutual understanding of how the allure can wear off if sex is treated too cheaply. Couples should maintain their sex lives with this knowledge. It's a cooperative effort. Plan for periods of sexual separation. Give your libido a chance to replenish itself.

RABBI SHMULEY

To avoid overfamiliarity in marriage and keep passion alive, the Jewish religion requires the husband and wife to be separated during the five days of her menstruation and the following seven nights. During this time there is no intimacy—no hugging, snuggling, or kissing and definitely no sex. At the end of this period, the wife takes a ritual bath, after which she reunites with her husband. The anticipation they felt while apart explodes in a passionate reunion. The reason for their separation is not because she is "unclean," as some might think, but to increase sexual desire so the marriage doesn't become boring due to easy availability.

There are many other ways to create unavailability as well. When you go to bed at night, keep your nightgown on and don't touch. Talk in bed rather than immediately watching TV. Have conversations about intimate subjects, and discuss topics that give you new insight into each other and that stoke the fires of desire. Let your words heighten attraction, and go to bed without touching. When you do touch, make out for an hour with lingerie or pajamas on. When you're physically apart, have long, sexy conversations.

Being unavailable will frustrate consummation, and your desire will grow. Flirting, teasing, sending love notes to one another, having erotic conversations—all of this fuels passion. Feel the arousal. Feed the anticipation. Let it simmer, draw it out, and take pleasure in it. Even in the act of lovemaking, take your time. Remove your clothes slowly. Give sensual massages before you even kiss. Make every move involve an obstacle, slowing you down, forcing you to engage your mind. Kiss the ears, elbows, knees, and hair. Let passion build slowly as you create a sensual connection that will continue even after the lovemaking is over. Remember, sex is to be cherished. It's magical. It's sacred.

CHAPTER 20

Mystery

It was from the difference between us, not from the affinities and likenesses, but from the difference, that that love came: and it was itself the bridge, the only bridge, across what divided us.

URSULA LE GUIN

E roticism is a journey to the unknown. It involves the deepest mysteries of our sexuality and our humanity. Where there's no mystery, there's no erotic discovery. Eroticism is a lurch in the shadows. It thrives on the unfamiliar. Curiosity, imagination, learning—these fuel our passions, stimulate our minds, and send currents of excitement through our bodies. When there's no mystery left in love and life, we become dulled. When we know everything about each other and think there's nothing new to discover together, our natural curiosity withers and the intensity of our love diminishes.

Pamela

In film and literature, there is a lot of romanticism about the age of exploration, the questing explorer setting off to discover the world. We enjoy this kind of story because it recreates a sense of darkness and the unknown. It gives us a sense of mystery that is absent in our daily lives. Mystery gives joy to life because it is still open to possibilities. When there is still mystery left in the world, our greatest hopes and greatest fears can still be just around the corner. We could find our life's love or the monsters of our nightmares. Even the things we are afraid of can give us something to strive against, something to give meaning and drama to our otherwise flat and featureless lives.

Contrast this with the world as we know it today, where every unexplored space has already been discovered, every corner of our planet mapped out, every creek or forest divided up and possessed. Our world has been demystified, but our minds still long for frontiers. We long for the feeling of wonder we felt as a child as we stared out at a new world, not yet sensible, that was full of fascinating things. The colorful mythologies of ancient cultures also show us this relationship between meaning and the unknown. We long to be like the first cultures as they huddled in their homes on the banks of rivers and heard the thunder above them and imagined gods fighting in the heavens. Think of how brilliant and bright and dangerous but wonderful the world was to them.

And so we invent the mystery that we lack. Our need for adventure and novelty and promise must be satisfied in literature and film and television. There we allow our imaginations to quest in unfamiliar landscapes. But what many of us do not realize is that there is still mystery and wonder to be found in all of our lives, and it is in the most obvious of places. When we spend a lot of time with someone, we often come to think that we know everything about them, that we have exhausted all of their mystery. But you never truly know a person: there is always more to your partner. If you think there isn't, that's because your relationship has become stuck in a monotonous routine, and you are looking in the same place every day for something new. Even a minor change of context can suddenly remind us that this other person, this many-faceted jewel, is still mostly unknown to us. Every lover is an undiscovered country. There are infinite depths in each of us, enough for a whole life's wandering. Together we can be explorers, questing into each other's soul and body, charting their reaches. It is love that is the final frontier.

Remaining open to these possibilities in each other is something you have to *do*: it doesn't just happen. It is something that must be cultivated in ourselves, and this is done by being open to the depths in ourselves too. It means constant development of ourselves, constant willingness to evolve and change and grow, to be the kind of dynamic person that can hold another's fascination. We should never stop learning or discovering new dimensions to ourselves, facets we never knew were there until an unexpected experience or a surprising new person unearthed them. It means never stopping making discoveries by going places we've never been, setting ourselves new challenges, standing up for causes we believe in, meeting interesting people, seeing the world through their eyes, and learning something new: painting, sculpting, drawing, writing, or mastering a new language.

This process of finding the depths within ourselves is impossible without another. The capacity of another person to surprise us, to reveal something new every day, is also a mirror in which we see greater possibilities in ourselves. In dialogue with another soul, our own soul deepens. We learn to see ourselves with another's eyes and see what they see in us. This is why the real joy of life is found in love with someone else. Not only do we discover someone else, but we learn that we too contain mysteries we could not even imagine. It is in this way that we can infuse our relationships—our lives—with mystery. It's in sexual intimacy that we can heal each other sensually, but to do this, we need mystery in our relationships.

We need to reach for more, like Jay Gatsby stretching out his arms toward the dark waters, trembling with anticipation, his eyes fixed on the green light of his soul mate's home. We need to lift our eyes from the tired "knowns" of life and look into the deep unknown—in the world, in each other, and within ourselves.

RABBI SHMULEY

The reason mystery is essential to erotic desires is that curiosity, this hunger for knowledge that is integral to being human, is the soul of life. To be alive is to learn, to seek, to know. This is the essence of sexuality, and it's the essence of life itself. In the Bible, the word to describe sex is *yediah*, which is knowledge. Adam *knew* his wife, and she conceived an offspring. This knowing goes far beyond sex—it means to comprehend, to understand, *to learn*. When God says in Exodus 6:7, "You shall know that I am the Lord your God," the word for *know* here is the same as that used for sexual knowledge. The intimate knowing between a man and woman is not only profoundly personal, but also dynamic. You are always learning, knowing, and understanding each other. People change and grow. There are layers to each of us, and we can spend a lifetime peeling them back to discover something new. Our desire needs to be fueled by this need to learn. It is ignited by mystery.

As we've discussed, Western sexuality is in a state of crisis today. Divorce is rampant, people aren't getting married, and pornography has led to a degradation of the sexual experience. We have become desensitized, restless, and deeply dissatisfied in our erotic relationships. The sexual revolution promised liberation, but it also delivered dysfunction. One of the main reasons for this decline is that Western sexuality is no longer based on knowledge. We aren't seeking to get to know someone, to understand them and connect with them emotionally, spiritually, and intellectually. We're focused only on the physical. We treat sex as a merely physical act driven by instincts and hormones rather than looking to connect with another person in the deepest way possible. Our goal is to purge ourselves of our sexual need—to sate our hunger and quiet our bodies—instead of taking the time and feeling the tension of deeper sensuality.

Embracing mystery and seeking knowledge is an unsettling journey for at least a couple of reasons. First, when we seek to know someone and to unlock all their mysteries, we have to give that person power over us. We are admitting to them we don't know everything, that we're ignorant. This takes humility and trust, which is disconcerting. Second, we don't know what we're going to discover when we start peeling back those layers. We feel anxious and nervous. But these feelings electrify us. They make us feel alive. They turn life into an adventure. This is the soul of erotic longing: You are mysteriously drawn to another person, so much so you need to find out everything about her (or him). You lie awake at night thinking about what you will discover when you talk to her again. You want to know what she thinks, how she will move when you touch her in a new way, the sound of her breathing when you kiss her, the sway of her body when she listens to a new song, the light in her eyes when she tastes a new flavor. You want to discover what she thinks of you, your thoughts, your feelings, how you perceive life and love. This intimate knowing means to experience the whole person, and its intensity is unsettling and even a little frightening.

Mystery keeps us on edge; our hearts beat a little faster with anticipation and anxiety. We know this simply by watching an Alfred Hitchcock film. The frightening journey that leads to Mrs. Bates's rotting corpse in *Psycho*. The anxiety of witnessing a possible murder in *Rear Window*. The mystery and sense of dread surrounding Maxim de Winter's first wife in *Rebecca*. The unknown stimulates the mind and imagination, making our fingers tingle as we breathlessly wait to discover what happens next.

Curiosity in any form quickens our blood and makes us feel alive: Learning the mysteries of science, art, and philosophy. Seeing the world through the eyes of someone completely different from ourselves.

Developing a new skill, unlocking our potential, opening ourselves up to others who can teach us and lead us down exciting paths we never knew were there. The erotic experience is infused throughout with this appetite for each other, this quest into each other's souls. The mechanical nature of sex between people who have become strangers to each other is the opposite of sex between two people who find vitality and fascination in the never-ending inquiry into each other. What is erotic about sex is that it is with another person, another mind, another soul. But it isn't easy. It takes courage, humility, and a willingness to participate in life instead of simply observing it.

The problem with Western sexuality is that it never wants to be unsettled. Our bodies have needs, they're sexually frustrated, so the goal is to release that buildup as soon as possible—masturbation, casual sex, porn, even disconnected sex with your partner. None of these things is wrong in itself, but the problem is that they are presented as viable alternatives to sexual experience by our culture: a need just like any other, a commodity for consumption. Just release and get it over so the ache is eased. No more discomfort. No more longing. No more desire. Sex puts an end to our hunger, which is why the orgasm is so central to sex today. We have sex to achieve climax instead of having sex to connect with another person, to get to know what excites them, to embark on a sensual journey together.

Mystery can't exist in a relationship that has no interest in a quest for knowledge. This is why sex dies off so quickly in a marriage. If sex is simply to satisfy hunger, then after a few years, if not sooner, not much hunger is left after eating the same dinner every night. Pretty soon you're going to want something else, and you'll start going to restaurants instead of staying home. But when sex has mystery, it's a completely different dynamic. You're making love because you want to know this person deeply and intimately. Your partner has infinite layers, and you want to peel each one back erotically. Instead of a destination, sex becomes an erotic journey of exploration.

This mysterious adventure is exciting and challenging because objects are put in the way of our desires. We have to strive and reach for what's beyond us. If it's predictable and right there in front of us, there's no mystery to it—there's no unknown. Obstacles frustrate the fulfillment of our sexual desire, and these are fundamental to eroticism. Erotic obstacles provide confirmation of our desirability, that someone will work hard and sacrifice much to have us—that makes us feel incredibly sexy and desirable.

Those obstacles can be any number of things—age, religion, living apart, and having different societal beliefs. All of these create tension because of unavailability, but when we allow erotic desire to move us, we can overcome anything. The younger man will defy social stigma to win the love of the older woman he desires. Two people who meet momentarily on vacation in Paris but live on opposite sides of the world will move heaven and earth to be together. Family commitments, religious dogma, socially imposed shame—none of it will stand in the way of true love and desire. When a man will fight for you, overcome great obstacles for you, sacrifice for you, your passion is kindled. You feel special, beautiful, worthy, and sexy. And this is part of the interplay between femininity and masculinity. The tension between the two sexes is highly erotic.

Eroticism needs obstacles to keep it alive. This is why pornography is so unsatisfying. There's no mystery, nothing standing in the way of fulfillment, nothing for the mind to discover. For something to be erotic, it can't be attained so easily that all thought is shut off. The mind must be engaged, thinking, imagining, anticipating. A woman's mind is much more alluring than her body, because its her mind that the man seeks to master, to discover, and to know. Her mind is the holy grail at the end of his quest.

We're not, of course, suggesting people withhold sex for just any reason; it's not about withholding, but about creating anticipation. We must learn to complement each other, to learn the nature of our partner's desires, to shape ourselves to them, and to engage all of our creativity to hold our love lives in a delicate balance of intimacy and distance. We must be the interesting, elusive, enigmatic people that our partners fell in love with. We must learn to always hold something in reserve, retaining some mystery. "Hate to sound sleazy," wrote Tupac Shakur, "but tease me. I don't want it if it's that easy."

We lose our allure to each other if we are wholly possessed by the other. We need to understand the need in our partners to always have something to want. It's not withholding; this is just how desire works. It would be neglect to ignore it. Sexiness always involves some kind of restraint—it is suffocated when everything is too free, too attainable. In sex, this can involve sensuality and playfulness—it varies for each couple, but for example, this is the essential appeal of sexy lingerie. It's sexy because it holds something back—it conceals at the same time as it reveals. To play with desire, to titillate, we have to understand that there must always remain something to strive for, something more to desire. Everything isn't out in the light. A couple can keep their flame alive by learning to tease each other with shadows and suggestion, an erotic glance or the lightest of touches. Curiosity is awakened, and the mind, not just the body, is engaged. When we see less, we are excited more by the possibilities. The sexual tension this creates is electrifying.

The commodification of sex in Western culture—accelerated and deepened by the digital age—has taken the mystery out of sex. It has also robbed us of intimacy because mystery is integral to intimacy. If every part of us, every aspect of our sexuality, is made public, there aren't any private spaces left to share intimate moments. This privacy isn't a physical space, but the private parts of ourselves. If everything we are is out there on full display—like so many young people have learned to do today through webcams, Snapchat, and sexting—there isn't anything secret left to share with our partners. This drive toward ever-greater exposure produces perverse outcomes: it puts everyone in competition with each other, pressuring us to focus exclusively on our appearance. It creates a cultural tendency toward narcissism and alienation and turns us away from finding satisfaction in our relationships. Our private lives, our intimate selves, our mysteries have become like a secret shared with too many people.

How do you bring back hiddenness? How do you maintain mystery in your long-term relationships? One of the first things you can do is develop your own sense of mystery. Learn more about the world, learn more about yourself. Grow and expand. Let your curiosity run wild. When it comes to sex, it is important to approach it with a sense of creativity and passion. Sometimes this means we don't bare everything. Each time should be a new experience, unlike before, a dance, or an opportunity to explore. Put on some lingerie, and tease your partner by hiding parts of yourself. Or allow yourself to be sexually forward, provocatively so, but in a completely unexpected context.

During times of sexual separation (as we talked about in the previous chapter), perhaps don't let your partner see you naked, or be selective about nudity. When you do have sex, don't always do it with the lights on or with mirrors on the walls revealing everything. Try making love in the dark or by soft candlelight or moonlight. Focus on your breathing. Slowly touch each other. Let your imagination, not just your body, take over. Use all your senses, not just your eyes. Allow mystery to set your erotic minds free. Celebrate each other through restraint and patient discovery. Think of your bodies not as a quick means to sexual gratification, but as something to discover, contemplate, and know in every detail. Explore, as Pablo Neruda writes in his poem "Ode to A Naked Beauty", the beauty in every line and curve.[2]

CHAPTER 21

Forbiddenness

There is a charm about the forbidden that makes it unspeakably desirable.

MARK TWAIN

M arriage can be boring. It's true. Long-term relationships become dull because of too much familiarity and complacency. The electrifying intensity of eroticism sputters out because imagination and exciting possibilities are abandoned for concrete realities and daily necessities. This can flatten our experience, deadening us

Experiencing the real peaks and troughs of life is part of living. I think about it: in the greatest literature it's always the great events—the triumphs and the tragedies—that we read about. This is because those are the things that stand out, those are the things that sustain interest. Sometimes it is a personal tragedy that knocks us out of our routine and allows us to truly see the world again, to experience it keenly, and to realize that we have had a veil over our eyes.

Anaïs Nin wrote in her diary that people who live in a sheltered, delicate world think they're living, but they're really not. They're merely existing, drifting on the still waters of safety and security. They think this is life.

Then something happens—they read a book or poem, see a film, take a trip, meet someone erotically compelling, experience the unexpected, or taste a bit of danger. Their pulse is quickened, their imagination awakens, and they realize they haven't been living; they've been hibernating:

> The symptoms of hibernating are easily detectable: first, restlessness. The second symp-
> tom (when hibernating becomes dangerous and might degenerate into death): absence
> of pleasure. That is all. It appears like an innocuous illness. Monotony, boredom,
> death. Millions live like this (or die like this) without knowing it. They work in offices.
> They drive a car. They picnic with their families. They raise children. And then some
> shock treatment takes place, a person, a book, a song, and it awakens them and saves
> them from death. Some never awaken. They are like the people who go to sleep in the
> snow and never awaken.[1]

Nin wrote that reality, the humdrum of life, didn't impress her. She believed in "intoxication, in ecstasy, and when ordinary life shackles me, I escape, one way or another. No more walls."[2]

Pamela

"No more walls!" is a cry of the soul living a narrow, scripted life. It's a primal and very human reaction. I often compare this sense of containment within our everyday lives to the experience of animals in industrial farming. Think of battery hens, each in tiny cages, or dairy cows, constricted in enclo-sures, forced simply to produce day in day out. It helps people understand the cruelty these animals undergo when it is related to our daily lives, but it also helps us understand the ways in which our lives can become cages for us, and this is the first step to escaping them. Even soul mates are little consolation to each other if their lives together are lived in a cage.

We aren't meant to live a finite life defined by the doldrums of duties and material pursuits. As spiritual creatures, we long for more.

We have imaginations that need to fly free. We hunger for new experiences to broaden and expand our existence. As much as we must live in a world of everyday realities, we need our minds to soar into the far reaches of possibilities—and we need our bodies to feel their electrifying effects.

When this happens, we are truly ourselves. We are living. Imagining a life beyond the one we have inspires us to *become* not simply *be*. Of course, if we let imagination completely take over, we'll be lost in a fantasy world. We need the balance of both—the securities of reality and the perils of fantasy. This is essential to our humanity. Not only do we need to feel the certainty of the earth beneath our feet, we also need to touch the infinite and feel its expanse in our spirits.

Imagination is essential to this freedom. It is the "medium of the process of infinitizing," Søren Kierkegaard wrote. "What feeling, knowledge, or will a man has, depends in the last resort upon what imagination he has. . . . For in order to be aware of oneself and God imagination must enable a man to soar higher than the misty precinct of the probable, it must wrench one out of this and, by making possible that which transcends the *quantum satis* of every experience, it must teach him to hope and fear, or to fear and hope."[3] When we remove adventure and imagination from our lives, we become stagnant. We lose a primal element of ourselves. We feel caged, surrounded by concrete walls. Our desire to be transcendent is tucked away under layers of daily duties. We aren't meant to live this way. We're meant to be free. "Freedom," as Rabbi Nachman of Bratslav said, "is a world of joy."

This freedom is often lost in marriage and long-term relationships because we're afraid to step beyond the lines that have defined our lives. These lines in marriage are drawn by familiarity and security within a monogamous relationship, but there's something else that turns these lines into walls—the legal construct of the marital union. Legalities are essentially boring because they minimize risk. Imagination—being open to possibilities, living out our fantasies, and seeking adventure, particularly in something that's forbidden—is fraught with risk. Everything we know about eroticism goes against the mundane and customary. We're excited and awakened when we feel the pulse of desire to experience something beyond the walls. It becomes a fever. We can't control it. It's powerful and wild.

The problem with marriage is that it is designed for domestication and comfort. We declare to an entire community that this is a legal relationship for security and children, if possible. Its purpose is to form ties that bind, ties that last, ties that are secure. There is great comfort in a marriage, but it can create restlessness. Being bound by a legal code incites us to want more, to break the rules, to look for excitement. Consider Adam and Eve in the Garden. They were perfectly happy, content, and secure, but there were rules. If they tasted the forbidden fruit, they would destroy their peaceful existence. And that's exactly what they did. What would possess them to risk everything to taste the forbidden fruit? Why would they give up their comfort and security? They needed to feel free, to expand beyond the constraints of the law, to soar beyond the finite and be limitless, to be god-like. That was the real temptation—to be infinite, like God. In a way she didn't intend, Mae West was right when she said, "To err is human—but it feels divine." It feels divine because we imagine we can be limitless like God. That glorious freedom is erotic.

The law creates a kind of tyranny over the mind. It makes us feel safe, but it can be oppressive. We hate to be oppressed. It flies in the face of humanity, which is naturally hostile to authoritarian control. To overcome tyranny, to grab hold of the forbidden fruit—to sin—is deeply erotic because it enlivens our primal selves. This is why adultery is so powerful. It feeds our inmost hunger. We want most what we cannot have. The attractive woman at the dance club who casts a glance a man's way is intoxicating until he finds out she's a prostitute. She's only in it for the money. There's nothing to win over, just a transaction to be made. Erotic attraction dies instantly.

In this example, the discovery that this potential new sexual partner is no longer off-limits in any way is deflating: a disappointment. It's a let down, not only because she's a sure thing, but because he doesn't feel as exciting as he did before. He's not forbidden *to her*. Forbiddenness is the core of eroticism because getting another person to cross boundaries for you—to risk everything for you—is the ultimate form of validation. If you can get someone to do something sinful, to push through the greatest obstacles to have you—even do something that violates their conscience and values for you, then you've got solid proof that you're pretty attractive. That's compelling! That's how special and desirable you are. That's why sin is so powerfully erotic. For someone to do something so extreme, to break vows to others, to potentially soil their own reputation, you must be the most exciting, amazing person in the world. To get what you're not supposed to have is the ultimate win, raising you above the rules, conferring a special status on you.

It's in pushing against obstacles that passion is found. This is where tension is created. If there's no boundary to cross, nothing forbidden—if everything is out in the open and safe, there's nothing to imagine having, no wanting, longing, desiring, hungering. This is the tension created by marriage. You're within a legal construct in which other people are forbidden. The more familiar and easily attainable your spouse becomes, the more passion fades and the more exciting other people outside the marriage become.

The marriage began with fire, but eventually—if efforts aren't made to keep it alive—it grows cold. This doesn't mean everyone cheats, but, as we've seen, many are unsatisfied in their long-term relationships. They feel something is missing. That missing piece is eroticism—the fire of desire. It is one of the cruelest things about how desire works—that when a relationship begins to express real dedication and commitment is also when, without the proper effort, it begins to lose its spark. Erich Fromm, in *The Art of Loving*, describes this well:

> *If two people who have been strangers, as all of us are, suddenly let the wall between them break down, and feel close, feel one, this moment of oneness is one of the most exhilarating, most exciting experiences in life. It is all the more wonderful and mirac- ulous for persons who have been shut off, isolated, without love. This miracle of sudden intimacy is often facilitated if it is combined with, or initiated by, sexual attraction and consummation. However, this type of love is by its very nature not lasting. The two persons become well acquainted, their intimacy loses more and more its miraculous character, until their antagonism, their disappointments, their mutual boredom kill whatever is left of the initial excitement.*[4]

Some would say this decline of passion in monogamous relationships is natural and inevitable. Evolutionary psychologists claim sex is all about procreation and survival of species, and as you get older, sex hormones decline, the sex drive fades, men suffer from erectile dysfunction, and women can't have children any longer. This, the scientists say, is your body telling you erotic passions are a thing of the past and now it's time to go quietly into that good night.

RABBI SHMULEY

Religion sometimes agrees with this sentiment. The Catholic Church has maintained that sex is primarily for procreation—when the time for making babies is past, sexuality may not matter as much. Not long after Viagra first came out, I was discussing with a priest whether this medicine was a good thing. The priest was against it because he believed that as we get older we should be freed of the sexual urge so we can dedicate ourselves to prayer, service, and family. I respectfully disagreed, replying, "In that case we should be opposed to dental implants. Our teeth wear down and we can't eat steak, so we should give up that desire and be satisfied with applesauce and devote our lives to less material and more spiritual pursuits." The point is that medical advances can help us achieve what is healthy for us. Sexuality and passion are healthy and part of who we are. That doesn't change when we grow older.

Still, many people do give up and lose their sexual passion. Life does get in the way. Marriage can be monotonous. Even when you're younger, you can lose interest in sex with the same person. Does this mean long-term relationships are doomed? Are we left with settling for a passionless marriage, committing adultery, or resorting to an open marriage where we invite other people into our sacred space and rob it of intimacy?

We don't believe it is. We believe the "sinful" impulses and "forbidden" qualities that make sex so erotic can be brought into marriage. The legal construct doesn't have to kill desire. Marriage doesn't have to be boring. The solution is to *make marriage "sinful."* Everyone has impulses that make them hunger for what they can't have. It's human to be excited by what's forbidden. That is especially true with sex. It would be unhealthy to deny these impulses—they're part of who we are. That's the problem in many of today's marriages. People deny their natural desires. They bury them deep so they no longer feel those deep adventurous, sometimes dangerous, urges. Shutting down these parts of ourselves—imagination, sinfulness, and the hope of possibilities outside the day-to-day routine—cools our desire for each other.

The solution isn't denying our natural desires. We need to express and share them, be free and explore them—but this can be done *without* giving expression to the destructive impulses of infidelity, which can ruin perfectly good marriages and relationships. It can be done *within* the legal structure of marriage, within a committed, monogamous relationship where love flourishes. We must constantly work at bringing into our marriages the elements of unavailability, mystery, and forbiddenness. But we need to keep our final goal in mind—the health and welfare of our marriage. Forbiddenness, or sinfulness, has to be kept within bounds because eroticism is fire. If you have a fire in your house to keep it warm, you have to maintain it and guard it to make sure it stays in the fireplace. You don't want it getting out of control and burning down the house.

How do you do this? How do you bring some forbiddenness into your relationship without it becoming destructive? One of the first things we suggest is for a wife to share her fantasies with her husband—this is particularly relevant if the husband has stopped seeing his wife as sexually desirable. If your husband thinks you're just a mother and housekeeper, he needs to see you in a new light—as a sexually compelling woman, as the woman he fell in love with and pursued. It's uncomfortable to do at first, but it works when you both understand your reason for doing it. Share all your fantasies, not only hidden sexual fantasies about your spouse, but fantasies about other people, including fantasies for strangers. You have them. They make you feel that tingle of excitement deep inside. Don't suppress them. Set them free, but not by acting out with a stranger. Share them with your husband. When you do, he will see you with new eyes and understand the depth of your irrepressible sexual longing. You will be giving him a peek into something secret, forbidden, and sinful. This will unnerve him and bring out some jealousy, but it will also stimulate his erotic desires. He will see you as the sexual creature you are, and he will want to possess you.

Most people believe they need to be proper in relationships. They want to pretend there are no wrinkles, that they're pure. But this isn't true. We all have transgressive erotic fantasy. Sharing our fantasies with each other is like turning a shirt inside out. We're inverting ourselves and showing all the seams. We can't be fully known by our spouse if there's no erotic danger in the relationship, if it's purged of all sinfulness. A sanitized marriage is a recipe for boredom. Bringing some fantasy forbiddenness into the relationship gives it the electric shock it needs. It brings excitement and passion back into our lives.

Some people might recoil at the thought of being so open with their spouse. They might think it's playing with fire, that it's best not to share forbidden desires—or even to think them. But that's just living in denial of who we are. One of the ways a man extinguishes his wife's sexuality is to see her only as a wife, not as a powerfully erotic woman who, in some ways, is forbidden to him. Men want a woman sexy in bed, but they fail to fan the flames because they want the security. They want the safety and comfort that marriage brings. But it's this delicate, easy life that kills passion. He needs to be willing to set his wife free. She needs to do the same for him.

This is hard to do. Stepping away from what's concrete and certain and entering the world of fantasy is scary. It's fraught with danger. It's a fire. But it doesn't have to become destructive. It can be contained within the relationship, giving it the heat of passion it needs. Nothing worthwhile can come about in love, without a little bit of risk. You have to have a stake in a relationship to get rewards from it. If we want love to work, then we have to work at it. That means taking risks, putting ourselves out there, and being vulnerable. If we don't, we'll become lazy and indifferent.

Bringing forbiddenness into a marriage is dangerous, but it works. In some cases, when a marriage is truly moribund, you have to give it shock treatment. Take your wife to a bar, but go in separately. Let her sit at the bar while you watch her from a distance. Watch her as if you were a stranger. Imagine she's not yours. Other men will begin to gravitate to her, talk to her, and her attractiveness will be on full display. This will both worry and excite you, and when you go home you will have passionate sex because you see her as something new. She's not just your wife; she's a mysterious woman, a "stranger." She's forbidden.

This can be difficult to do, as can sharing fantasies about strangers. It challenges trust. When she tells you she's attracted to other men, part of you doesn't trust her—that's because human nature isn't trustworthy, especially if it has been neglected. But if you have a great passionate sex life together, she won't stray. It's not that she isn't tempted, but she makes a conscious choice not to because she can have amazing, fulfilling sex in the marriage, all the more pleasurable because its joined to intimacy. Other men have nothing to offer her. Your trust then is in the principles of a relationship not in her human nature. A relationship is supposed to be satisfying and pleasurable. If it is, a person will want to stay in the relationship because they're getting what they want—they're being fulfilled.

The greatest defense against infidelity is erotic satisfaction within marriage. When you make the relationship a little sinful, you inoculate it against actual transgression. You maintain your desire for each other instead of being warm and cozy "friends" and lusting after someone else. Sharing fantasies and pretending to be a stranger aren't the only ways to do this. Every couple needs to find out what works best for them. Whatever it is, it needs to have a sense of danger to it. It needs to be a little naughty.

Pamela

A huge part of the art of sensuality involves becoming attuned to every exquisite detail of the experience, for example, during a date, attending to textures, sounds, and tastes. You become more aware of your body, more aware of your partner's body, their posture, their body language. The sense of place and time. All of the minutiae. The variation, the little fluctuations, the ebb and flow of conversation, the ambient noise: the immediacy of all of this, it heightens sensation and gives everything a deeply erotic subtext—an experience I describe in a poem called "Dinner Date":

> Sit across from each other
> The Tease
> The Dance
> The eye contact without touching
> Look at each other

Look at everything

Ankles, legs

Neck

Mouth

How they move, walk

How they talk with others

Observe the scene

Smell the air between you

The flowers, the bees

The food

Taste every bite

Think of the textures...

what you touch

The glass

The fork

The linen between your fingers

The roots of your hair

Your own skin

Think of the person nude

Fantasize

That you are on his lap

or under the table.

Awaken mystery by going out to a restaurant with friends and touching your partner under the table. Your spouse has to pretend like it's not happening and keep the feelings you're awakening under control. By the time you get home, you'll be ripping each other's clothes off. Your desire and lust will be set free, not by an illicit lover, but by your spouse.

Meet at a hotel during work as if you're having an affair. Read erotic literature to each other and play out fantasies. Buy some sex toys together; experiment and push each other's boundaries. Have phone sex. Take erotic pictures of yourself and send them to your spouse. Go on business trips together and have a secret liaison at an exotic hotel. Find new places to make love. Discover new ways to excite each other, and the more sinful within the framework of your marriage, the better. Sexual attraction is enhanced by forbiddenness because the mind gravitates toward forbidden things like nothing else. Let it go, but make the journey together.

CHAPTER 22

Vertical Discovery

I love thee to the depth and breadth and height
My soul can reach, when feeling out of sight
For the ends of being and ideal grace.

ELIZABETH BARRETT BROWNING

E lizabeth Barrett lived most of her life alone, sickly and under her father's control. She never thought she would find love or, more likely, that anyone would love her. This changed at the age of forty when Robert Browning asked to meet her. She had become a successful poet (rare for a woman at that time), and he was interested in her work. Their first meeting launched one of the greatest courtships recorded in literature.

Robert and Elizabeth were prolific letter writers, corresponding continuously as they were often apart. Because her father disapproved of the relationship, their courtship was secret and they were forced to elope. Elizabeth's father eventually disinherited her. She and Robert lived happily together despite the family conflict, writing poetry, making friends with artists and writers, traveling when her health allowed it. They had one son together, but her health continued to be poor and she died in 1861 in her husband's arms. Robert said she passed away peacefully with a smile. The last word on her lips was "Beautiful."

The letters between Robert and Elizabeth have survived and reflect a depth of intimacy rarely experienced in our frenzied, often shallow, and materialistic times. Their correspondence reveals two people who had the courage and trust to share their innermost selves with each other. They weren't afraid to pull back the veil for the other to peer within. They wrote about everything: politics, literature, poetry, theology, and everyday concerns. Mostly, they spoke of their love, sprinkling their letters with personal experiences so they could live as one, even though they were apart. Through heartfelt and intelligent communication, they grew to intimately know each other. Never satisfied to live on the surface, they dove into the depths and found beauty behind the eyes of the other. With a shared vulnerability, their marriage remained steadfast and true.

Elizabeth's famous poem "How Do I Love Thee?" captures the essence of what love means:

> *How do I love thee?*
> *Let me count the ways.*
> *I love thee to the depth and breadth and height*
> *My soul can reach, when feeling out of sight*
> *For the ends of being and ideal grace.*
> *I love thee to the level of every day's*
> *Most quiet need, by sun and candle-light.*
> *I love thee freely, as men strive for right.*
> *I love thee purely, as they turn from praise.*
> *I love thee with the passion put to use*
> *In my old griefs, and with my childhood's faith.*
> *I love thee with a love I seemed to lose*
> *With my lost saints.*
> *I love thee with the breath,*
> *Smiles, tears, of all my life; and, if God choose,*
> *I shall but love thee better after death.*[1]

It's more than material interests or physical attraction. It's "depth and breadth and height." It's spiritual and profoundly erotic. Robert and Elizabeth's poetry and the letters they shared exude eroticism because their relationship had sensual intensity. "You are entirely what I love," Robert wrote to his "Ba," as he called her. "Not just a rose plucked off with an inch of stalk, but presented as a rose should be, with a green world of boughs around: all about you is 'to my heart'—to my mind, as they phrase it."[2]

Elizabeth taught him that the sweetness and power of love come from knowing another person completely. It's not just getting to know their physical form or sharing a life of routine responsibilities. It's more than just the "blossom of the rose." It's seeing a rose in its fullness—"how sweet it might become with superadded memories of the room and the chair and the vase, and the cutting stalks and pouring fresh water."[3]

Their letters are a story of two people on a quest—a journey to see one another's true form, and they never grew weary of discovering it. Whether it was a new poem one had written, a new experience and perspective on life, or something ordinary, like Elizabeth telling Robert how flowers he had sent to her made her feel—each word, each paragraph is a guidepost to the movements of her inner being:

> *Dearest, your flowers make the whole room look like April, they are so full of colours . . . growing fuller and fuller as we get nearer to the sun. The wind was melancholy too, all last night—oh, I think the wind melancholy just as you do,—or more than you do perhaps for having spent so many restless days and nights close on the seashore in Devonshire. I seem now always to hear the sea in the wind, voice within voice! But I like a sudden wind, not too loud,—a wind which you hear the rain in rather than the sea—and I like the half cloudy half sunny April weather, such as we have it here in England, with a west or south wind—I like and enjoy that; and remember vividly, how I used to like to walk or wade nearly up to my waist in the wet grass or weeds, with the sun over head, and the wind darkening or lightening the verdure all round.*[4]

Robert was to Elizabeth her "own especial fairy-tale," and she hoped he would never tire of their correspondence, even though at times, in speaking of their love and life, she worried he would get bored. "How one writes and writes over and over the same thing," she wrote. "But day by day the same sun rises over, and over again, and nobody is tired. Shall you ever tell me in your thoughts, I wonder, to get out of your sun?"[5]

His response was immediate and without doubt. He could never tire of her or her letters. Boredom held no place in their lives. She captivated his heart, mind, and soul. Knowing her was what he wanted most, and he wanted to be worthy of that knowledge. "I know I want every faculty I can by any possibility dare," he wrote. "I want all, and much more, to teach me what you are my own Ba, and what I should do to prove that I am taught, and do know."[6]

The Brownings maintained a passionate marriage because they understood the most important element in keeping love and desire alive: vertical discovery and renewal—going deeper and higher with the same person, plunging into the depths of who they are and flying to new heights. They never got bored with each other because they knew how to peel back the layers to discover something new and beautiful.

Couples get bored in long-term relationships because they explore each other horizontally—skimming the surface. It's a physical, immediate, and finite way of knowing. They get to know each other's bodies and what they're doing day to day. This can quickly become boring as they think they've discovered everything there is to know about the other person. They have no curiosity, no interest, so their minds and hearts often stray. They want to make new discoveries, but they believe there are none in the rote familiarity of their marriage.

As described in previous chapters, there are many ways to keep passion alive in long-term relationships—exploring mystery together, maintaining a sense of unavailability, and injecting some sinfulness into sex and intimacy. But these aren't enough, and they're certainly not the ultimate key to eroticism. None of these methods will work if there is no vertical discovery. There are only so many sexual positions to try, only so many restaurants to visit together, only so many trips to new places we can take. Eventually, we grow restless because the person we're with has become one-dimensional.

Human beings are not just a flat plane. We are complex with multiple levels to our being, and the really interesting parts are those within— our minds, our imagination, our creative insights. Here is where we find meaning, novelty, and connection. We crave intimacy with others because we want to know how they work. This desire for knowledge is the most important ingredient in any healthy relationship. As along as two people still want to know each other, their relationship is strong. They're still peeling off the layers—both in terms of clothing and their minds. But the moment they think they have exhausted knowledge of each other, the relationship has functionally terminated.

Our relationships die when we think we've got the other person all figured out. Inquisitive questions like those we pose at the beginning of a relationship cease. We don't ask about each other's dreams. We don't even ask about what happened at the office that day. We aren't curious about what our partner wants sexually; we do the same things we've been doing for the past ten years with no communication about what we long for or want to do differently. We stop wanting to taste every thoughtful morsel that falls from the other's table. Instead, we turn into potatoes, watching television every night instead of spending time talking. We tire of each other too quickly.

The reason for this is that we focus on horizontal discovery to find passion and excitement in life. We become restless, so we look for new "things" to distract us. We get tired of where we live, so we move. We get bored with our jobs, so we quit. We become restless, so we travel, planning one vacation after another. We're bored on the weekends, so we go to the mall and shop, buying new things we don't need. We're excited about the novelty for about a day or two, but then it passes and the rest-lessness resumes.

We become bored and agitated because horizontal renewal is never satisfied. We're just adding new things to our lives that will eventually bore us, forcing us to start the miserable cycle all over again. This is why material, horizontal distractions are so addicting. Pornography can be addictive because it doesn't satisfy our deepest sensual needs. It involves an initial "hit," which then quickly wears off, and there is an instant need to go back for more. The same is true with becoming addicted to shopping or to work. We hunger for more—uncontrollably—but we're never filled.

Contrast this to what the Brownings discovered—that spiritual connection keeps our love alive. We quiet our restlessness by discovering the deeper layers of life, beauty in unexpected places, ways of looking at others and existence from a new perspective. Gradually, we scrape away the outside of things and reveal their inner dimensions. We discover their essence. We don't try to overcome boredom by buying things, traveling, working, entertaining, or having an affair with a new body. Rather, we find the undiscovered sparks of life in our own backyard and our own bedroom; we find them in ourselves.

In the mid-fifties, Allen Ginsberg wrote a poem called "Sunflower Sutra" while traveling with Jack Kerouac. The poem begins with the two sitting on a dock near a railway yard under the shade of an old locomotive. Industrialization had plowed over nature, the desolation casting a gray shadow across "the gnarled steel roots of trees of machinery."[7] Kerouac points to a dead sunflower that extends from the earth as if part of the steel around it. Ginsberg is captivated by it. Even with all the soot and withered roots robbing the sunflower of its glory, Ginsberg saw its true form:

Poor dead flower? when did you forget you were a flower?[8]

Ginsberg then takes the skeleton flower and puts it to his side and pours out his poetic thoughts to Jack and anyone who will listen. "We're not our skin of grime," he declares. "We're golden sunflowers inside."[9]

With its obvious focus on the dehumanizing effects of industrialization, this poem has much to say about looking deeper into who we are: remembering our true selves. How many people in marriages are like the sunflower of Ginsberg's poem? How many once-vibrant crowns are now battered, their lives bleak and dusty? How many feel the grime of life on their skin, suffocating their relationships and their love? Too many, we believe. They have let the demands and distractions of a desensitized, materialistic world define who they are as individuals and as a couple. They have forgotten their true form. Failing to live vertically, they have succumbed to a horizontal existence—one that emulates the posture of death instead of life.

Those who embrace vertical renewal are awake and living a colorful life full of vitality. But those who insist on living horizontally, focusing on the here and now, the material things, on the physicality of sex alone, aren't truly living; they're merely surviving on things. They've allowed technology to rob them of their humanity. They've become mechanical instead of living sensually, and their relationships are suffering. They work hard, driving themselves to obtain material accumulations, but they've neglected their spirituality. This has led to an ethos of insecurity, fear, and apathy.

Boredom is the destroyer of life. It drives individuals to despair, it kills marriages, and it disconnects children from their families. Boredom causes us to make bad choices or to act out simply because we want to be titillated. The Talmud sums this up best: "When you have nothing to do, you do what you ought not to do." When we fail to see that there's more to life than the material, that we are more than what we produce, what we do, and what we see on a screen, we fade, like the sunflower dulled by soot. Life loses its mystery and wonder. The colors of the sunset and sunrise lose their vibrancy. The food we eat tastes bland. Books sit by our bedside unread. Questions that poured from us as children recede. Even sex bores us. We're no longer interested or curious. We look across the dinner table at the person we once thought was the most interesting in the world and we see a blank canvas, no splash of color, no interesting shapes and contours to examine, no exciting unknown work of art that makes our heart skip beats.

A relationship in trouble can place us in the worst kind of stasis. It's not just that an individual is experiencing boredom or depression with their life. When that happens, at least when the mood changes, it only takes one person to lift you out of it: yourself. When a relationship falls into the doldrums it is much harder to climb out, because you have to work together. If one person has the will but the other doesn't then it doesn't work. And knowing this weighs heavier on both people, detracting from all other pursuits, flattening our experience. Curing this malaise takes something powerful, something that moves us at the core of our being, and that remedy is erotic desire.

Eroticism is the desire to explore and discover the mysteries of life, to understand the complexities of our existence. The erotic is a magnetic pull toward the hidden essence of existence. It invites us to dive into the deep waters of life, to discover its mysteries. It's the draught of curiosity, mystery, and passion.

RABBI SHMULEY

We are infinite spiritual beings, and we can never be truly known if we ignore our spiritual natures. Proverbs calls the human spirit—the *Neshamah*—the *"lamp of the Lord that sheds light on one's inmost being."*[10] Our spirit is the essence of who we are. It is the seat of our thoughts, feelings, desires, and affections. If we are to know one another, we have to travel deep within—beyond the physical. This is God's gift to humanity—*"the Lord God formed man of the dust of the ground, and breathed into his nostrils the breath of life;*

and man became a living soul."[11] It's how we know another—it's the light that guides us as we search the dark depths of our souls.

There is an undiscovered world within each of us, and when we're in a long-term relationship, the thrill is exploring it and experiencing the novelty of it. When a man is erotically charged about a woman, he wants to know her in every way, not just sexually. How she breathes. What she's thinking. The shades of her hair. When they make love, he doesn't think about other women. Instead he peers into her eyes to penetrate her soul. Without speaking, they communicate. With a single glance, they feel powerful emotions that could never be captured by words.

A relationship is a living thing, and it lives through us. It cannot have life if *we* do not embrace life, if we do not *live* rich and interesting lives, constantly developing ourselves. We cannot see the depths in our partners if we do not explore the depths in ourselves. A shallow person can only see shallowly. Vertical discovery is reciprocal.

We live in a world that makes vertical discovery very difficult. Because everything is so fast paced, we don't take the time to talk, to write letters to one another, to reflect on nature and ourselves. Our focus is on gaining material goods instead of becoming better, more interesting, more knowledgeable people. Particularly in America, our superficial culture accounts for so many broken relationships because the individuals within those relationships are shallow, their connections flimsy, their inner being empty. Nothing can really compensate for the void inside us. We can try to stuff it with all the experiences and material goods in the world, but since it's a bottomless pit, we won't ever be able to fill it. We'll just keep feeding it, but it will never be satisfied. After a while, we become a prisoner to materialism, to those external experiences and objects we gather around us that leave us empty.

If we want our relationships to experience vertical renewal, we have to have vertical renewal within ourselves. If we don't, our relationships won't last. The greatest works of art—those by Michelangelo, Rembrandt, Velázquez, Caravaggio—have an eternal quality because they have depth. Superficial things don't last. Velvet art in plastic frames sold along highways doesn't endure the test of time. It has no profundity, no real significance. Relationships that last are more like Cézanne's *Mont Sainte-Victoire* than a neon Elvis on blue velvet. That's because the individuals within those relationships seek to be more than just shallow, material creatures surviving on the scraps of life. They study, read, meet new people, learn new skills. Everyone is infinite within, but too many are stunted because they've closed off that part of themselves. They've stopped learning and being curious. When they open themselves up, they grow, and their roots reach far into the rich soil. This strengthens relationships because they have become a person of depth, making vertical renewal possible.

The path to vertical renewal is best started when we're young, not when we're old and set in our shallow, dreary ways. If parents simply park their children in front of a screen, rarely interact with them, and never expose them to works of art, interesting places, or new experiences that broaden their horizons, they will only know horizontal renewal. If we give our children everything they want, showering them with material things, turning their eyes always toward the finite instead of the infinite, they will not grow to become people who long to explore the depths and heights of themselves and others.

Pamela

Most importantly, we need to allow children to be free to learn to use their senses, to be willing to examine new things without fear holding them back, and to step into the shadows where scary things dwell. Instead of hovering over them and directing them in everything they do, let them live curiously. Let them watch the world around them, including you. Set the example of what it means to live a vertical life full of confidence and sensuality. "What we do in this culture, which is a mistake, is to follow the children around," *said Jean Liedloff, author of* The Continuum Concept. "I advise people who are at the end of the 'in-arms' phase, when their infants start to creep, and then crawl, and then walk, to go about their own business doing useful, interesting things in and around the house."[12] *Don't just sit around in front of a computer, she says, be active:*

> Do the things that any reasonable hunter/gatherer would do like cooking, or gardening, or housework, or talking and laughing with your friends—things that a young child can see some kind of sense in. This way the child can follow you and watch you, which is the way nature intended. Then inevitably they will want to imitate you and help you. You don't have to ask them. They will automatically want to participate in the life that is unfolding around them, and they will naturally begin to move toward independence, just like any animal.[13]

Liedloff advises to teach children how to experience a passionate life. "What people really want, if it doesn't sound too soppy, is to live their love," *she says.* "Every day! Eat things because they love them, share food because they love to be with people. Just live out of love, love for beauty, love for truth, love for children and animals. It is our nature to live expansively and generously, not cautiously and calculatingly. The opposite of love is fear, not hate."[14]

If we raise children this way, they will live a life of vertical renewal, they will be in touch with themselves and the world around them. They'll experience what it feels like to be truly alive. In "Ladysmith," I describe what it's like to be aware of the sensuality of nature:

> The soft sounds . . .
> The crunching of wet grass . . . ,
> A frog's banter.

The sand squeaks

beneath my feet—

She stares at me

as . . .

I glide by her nest . . .

I wont hurt you...

Every step—means well,

A gentle touch, from the

leaves of a branch.

The feeling you get—

near cool wet pine . . .

The smell of that familiar boat dock.

The taste

Left anchored—the salty sea—

remembers me—

the . . . drawn waterways,

the long dragging stick follows . . .

Tracing . . .

so, you know where I've been.

In voluptuous circles,

wandering

. . . to heaven, and back.

Somewhere in the middle—I lay . . .

Eventually . . .

to watch the stars.

A man's smoky flannel over an old favorite bikini.

This is the kind of open awareness we want to pass on to our children—a curiosity of the world and a willingness to engage in it, to explore the fullness of nature and other people.

We become caught in a horizontal way of life when we allow, as Liedloff said, fear to overcome our love. Children who are kept from exploring and allowing their curiosity to roam because their parents are too afraid they'll fall and skin their knees will learn their parents' fear. That fear travels with them into their relationships. It takes courage to be open and vulnerable, to walk into unknown places. Allowing another person access to our inner world is intimidating. Often, we don't even want to know what's inside of us—especially when it comes to sexuality. We lack self-awareness. We hide from ourselves, refusing to explore the dark impulses within. We stay on the surface, splashing in the sunlit waters, too afraid to dive deep where the sunlight doesn't reach. But that is where we need to go, and it takes courage to do it.

It also takes trust. Reading through the Brownings' love letters, you can see the bond of trust they shared. To become emotionally vulnerable to another, to share your insecurities, your dreams, your weaknesses, your fantasies requires faith that the other person will not abuse you or shatter the glass heart you have entrusted to their care. We keep so many things guarded because we're afraid of getting hurt, but love drives out fear. If we want to live an erotic life and have a lasting relationship full of mystery, novelty, forbiddenness, and vertical renewal, we need to be fearless. When we're fearless, our life and our love expand, reaching into the depths and heights where the infinite dwells.

Part Six

PUTTING PASSION INTO PRACTICE

Our purpose in writing this book is primarily to achieve one thing: help couples connect more intimately and sensually, have better sex, form closer, more passionate relationships, and lead happier, more complete lives. This final section will provide some specific steps on how to do that, based on the pillars of eroticism: unavailability, mystery, forbiddenness, and vertical discovery. They may seem challenging, a little uncomfortable, even counterintuitive, but they will help turn those embers into flames.

Learning to Make Love

A good orgasm is satisfying, but a great orgasm can be a revela-
tion of your deepest being, unfolding the truth of who you are in
ecstatic communion with your lover.

DAVID DEIDA

In this modern age, especially in Western culture, we have often forgotten how to make love. The orgasm has been the focus instead of
sensuality, intimacy, and spiritual connection. Here are some practical
tips on how to make love in a way that will strengthen your relationship and
keep desire alive.

1. Practice having sex together in the tantric tradition, stopping
   short of full intercourse, for an entire week. Reexperience
   not just the pleasures of foreplay and long, sexual massages
   and intimate kissing, but also the erotic thrill of delayed
   gratification. This takes discipline, but it will bring you to the
   heights of passion and eroticism. All day, you'll be burning
   with desire for each other because release hasn't happened.
   These are the ideal periods to have phone sex with each
   other, even if it's just for a few minutes at a time. Practice
   heightening and maintaining your state of arousal. During this
   time, you'll see that you don't even notice strangers around

you. You will be intent on your spouse and the passion you're building together. Explore the world of Tantra together, where you learn that sexuality is not simply *doing* something with another person, but *being* present.

2. Stop being sexual and learn to be sensual, this is especially true for men. When making love, stop rushing to the finish line. Make sure you're touching and pleasuring each other for at least thirty minutes before sex. Start with making out with your clothes on, and then take them off slowly, kissing every part of skin along the way. Take your time. Learn to indulge all your senses in lovemaking.

3. Spend time kissing. Do it for up to an hour. Kissing creates intimacy and fuels desire. It's exchanging life breaths, giving you a glimpse into what it's like to be one soul. Prolonged kissing gives sex a different texture. It's more intimate, and its effects last longer.

4. Tap into sexual abandon by telling your wife to be loud. A man wants to hear his wife vocally express her yearning. She might feel self-conscious, but articulating sound increases desire and abandonment.

5. During sex, ask your husband what he wants you to do to him. Unleash his inner animal. Let him express what he wants. Join him in his own private fantasy world. If he's hesitant to tell you, make suggestions. Soon he'll respond as passion overwhelms him. Husbands can do the same thing for his wife. Get to know each other, communicate, and be open about what you want and enjoy.

6. Men, make sure your wife climaxes first. Too often men only think about themselves in sex and forget to meet the needs of the woman. This shuts down a woman's sexuality, and it robs the man of watching her succumb to pleasure. Instead,

husbands should put their wives first. Watch her get excited as you touch her in a dark movie theater. Do it discreetly, but feel the sexual tension and the excitement of pleasuring her.

7. Give each other long sensual massages that don't lead to sex or sensual release. Focus on every erogenous zone and let the passion build.

8. Once a week, take a bath or long shower together. Focus more on the soothing aspect than the erotic. Light candles. Learn to comfort each other and wash away the anxieties of life.

9. If you have a television in the bedroom, don't overindulge. There is no greater obstacle to a couple's intense sex life than the television. Put away the iPads and iPhones where you watch movies. Lessen the electronics in the bedroom and focus on each other, flesh and blood.

10. Mix up the locations where you have sex. Do things that heighten your awareness of everything around you. Drive to an empty golf course late at night and make love on the green. If there's a road nearby, every passing headlight will increase the thrill. Of course, don't get arrested! Be discreet and private. But be forbidden in your marriage.

11. Try herbal potions that enhance desire or use lotions to heighten an erotic response. If you get them off the Internet, make sure they're safe and backed up by medial authorities. It's the experimentation and novelty these provide that you want to focus on. Even if they don't work, use your imagination and make them work.

12. Abstain from masturbation and other forms of sexual self-gratification that lessen your sexual dependence on your spouse. Reduce the sexual outlets (mental, verbal, or otherwise) that you're exposed to and channel all your sexual

energy toward your partner. Show and feel desire only for your spouse. This will make your spouse come alive. Your desire has the power to make your spouse become a new person. When you diminish your hunger by releasing your sexual desires elsewhere, this power is reduced.

13. Don't compare your spouse mentally to other people. Learn to be subjective, not objective, in your attraction. Get images of supermodels, actresses, or the woman at the office out of your mind. Don't set up some unattainable ideal for your wife, which leads to disappointment. See her for herself. You chose her for a reason. Let her become your ideal, the only woman in your heart and mind. You can't be passionate about someone you find boring, especially if you're always comparing her to someone else. It's not fair to her, and it leaves you unsatisfied. If you want to bring passion back into your marriage, stop imposing objective standards on your wife and see her for the beautiful, passionate, and sexual person she is (the same goes for the wife about her husband). Everyone wants to feel special. If we don't feel special, we don't feel loved, and the passionate connection we long for will be broken.

Building Connection

Let me not to the marriage of true minds
Admit impediments. Love is not love
Which alters when it alteration finds,
Or bends with the remover to remove
O no! it is an ever-fixed mark
That looks on tempests and is never shaken;
It is the star to every wand'ring bark,
Whose worth's unknown, although his height be taken.
Love's not Time's fool, though rosy lips and cheeks
Within his bending sickle's compass come;
Love alters not with his brief hours and weeks,
But bears it out even to the edge of doom.
If this be error and upon me prov'd,
I never writ, nor no man ever lov'd.

SONNET 116

WILLIAM SHAKESPEARE

Disconnection within a long-term relationship is painful. You're joined together with another person but share no intimacy. You have union without communion. The marriage withers because it's not being maintained. This can lead to despair because people think they're locked into a dead relationship. They wonder how they can possibly go on. The future looks so bleak. Maybe they should get a divorce, or at least cheat so they don't feel so dead inside. Neither are good options—even the most seemingly hopeless cases can transform into something wonderful.

This point is well made in an old Jewish story about a man who complained to his rabbi that he was miserable in his marriage—the advice the rabbi gave was life changing:

"She's mean and harsh and demanding," [the man] lamented. "She serves me terrible food when she cooks at all. She does nothing but yell at me with a tongue like a shrew's. My life with her is a misery," moaned the man, "but I can't stand the scandal of a divorce. I hate to admit it, but I have actually been praying that she should die and leave me in peace." The wise Rabbi had a novel suggestion. "You know," he told his unhappy congregant, "when you make a pledge to charity and then do not fulfill the pledge before Rosh Hashanah, it's known that those close to you are liable to die in heavenly retribution. Why don't you make a large pledge to the community charity fund, and then not pay it?" The unhappy husband, a wealthy man not renowned for his generosity to communal causes, was delighted with the suggestion and implemented it immediately. He publicly pledged a large amount to the communal coffers, and then refused all attempts to collect the donation.

Months passed and the man eagerly awaited his wife's demise, but she appeared healthier than ever. The man became nervous and went to see the Rabbi. "Nothing is happening," he reported. "She doesn't even have the sniffles!" the Rabbi stroked his beard. "The death of a loved one is meant to be a punishment. Perhaps," he said, "you should make some efforts to appear to love her so that the divine decree will seem just. You have to create some evidence for the heavenly angels who will carry out the decree. Give her some gifts, compliment her, that sort of thing." The anxious husband was mollified. He set out for his home with renewed hope, ready to do his part. On the way, he passed the jeweler's shop and stopped in to buy his wife a lovely bracelet. She received the gift with astonishment, as he had not given her anything in many years. That night she served him his favorite supper.

Time went on and the man continued to invest himself in the project of appearing to love his wife so she would be punished by heaven with death. He complimented her, bought her gifts, and showered her with attention. In turn she stopped speaking to him harshly and began to treat him as a king of his palace. The months flew by in an ever happier whirlwind. Before he knew it, the man looked at the calendar and realized that it was almost Rosh Hashanah! He ran to the Rabbi in a panic and told him he was terrified that something would happen to his lovely wife! "You don't want her to die?" asked the Rabbi. "God forbid!" said the man. "We've never been more in love! She brings me infinite happiness." "In that case," said the sage, "you have no choice but to make good on your pledge!" The man paid his generous pledge, and the couple lived the proverbial happily ever after.[1]

The same story could be told of a wife who is unhappy in her marriage. Think of what could happen to your relationship if you work to create evidence of the love you have for each other? When you stop looking outside your marriage and focus on each other, you might find that your relationship isn't as bad as you think. Too often, we neglect the ones we love because we allow a materialistic, shallow culture to distract us from what's really important. If you truly want change, one of the first things you must do to create passionate connectedness in your marriage is to actually *focus on your marriage*. Pay attention to your spouse and give them what they need, instead of focusing on what you don't have and on your own needs. If you feel as if your relationship is dead, create the spark that will ignite passion once again. Instead of dropping out, tune in and turn on. This takes work, effort, and time, but it's worth it. When you start tending to your own garden, the beauty that grows there will surprise you.

Being Jealous

*I am jealous of this stocking...because it does what I can't.
Kisses your whole leg. And I'm jealous of this button.... It's with
you all day. I'm not.*

GRAHAM GREENE

Jealousy is usually seen as a negative, but the truth is a little bit of jealousy is essential in relationships. If you're never jealous, you must not think your spouse is attractive to others or has no sensual nature or sexual appeal another would find attractive. A little jealousy indicates there's eroticism inherent in your relationship. This inkling of distrust isn't aimed at your spouse—you trust her commitment and love for you. Your jealousy is rooted in the reality of her nature as a sexual creature who needs passionate connectedness to feel alive.

Noticing and accepting the fact that your spouse is attractive to others isn't easy. But it's necessary to keep passion in a marriage. If you begin to see your spouse as a nonsexual creature, intensity will die. So, it's important to both trust your partner and be jealous. This is a delicate balance to maintain. You need trust in your marriage, but there also has to be some measure of insecurity. This comes from the fact that your spouse is a sexual creature and attractive to others. This possibility makes you want to do everything you can to keep her. If you neglect your spouse, you will leave her tempted by the attentions of others. She will look outside the marriage for validation. But when you're jealous, you send a message to your spouse that she is valuable. If you're not jealous, you're saying you don't care, or you don't think she's sexually attractive enough to be wanted by another.

When it comes to long-term relationships, we want two things out of the same person. We look to our partners for stability—for love, trust, and devotion. At the same time we want passion, excitement, and desire. The comfortable nature of trust can squelch desire because you become bored. With predictability, there's no thrill of the chase.

The solution is to maintain a certain degree of healthy jealousy in your relationship so you don't relegate your partner to the status of a nonsexual being—one who fails to fill you with burning desire. This must be done without undermining trust. A serious breach in trust caused by infidelity destroys the foundation of the relationship. Rarely is it repaired. When your spouse rejects you, it confirms your own insecurities that maybe you're really not good enough, maybe in the final analysis you don't matter. This is why trust is so important to a marriage. Without it, the marriage breaks apart. But jealousy must also be present, because without it there's no fire to keep the passions burning.

These two coexist in a marriage through a creative tension that's achieved through radical honesty and openness. This is how you bring the balance of trust and jealousy into the relationship. You're honest about your spouse's inherent sexuality and attractiveness and how this causes you to distrust her on a natural, not moral, level. You know she is committed to you, and you to her, but her natural sexuality makes her desirable to others. This is why you must continually work to keep her and woo her. She needs to know that you think she is worth the struggle. Being honest about this fear, while being committed to the relationship, creates a healthy tension that is deeply erotic.

Channeling Your Femininity

To have her here in bed with me, breathing on me, her hair in my mouth——I count that something of a miracle.

HENRY MILLER

Putting passion into practice means cultivating sensuality and sexiness. Here are some tips on how women can ignite desire in their husbands.

1. Show your husband authentic appreciation. Praise your husband for everything he does for you and your family. Even when you're struggling or if you don't think he has done all he should, look for the silver lining and praise him. Compliments matter. Words can create their own reality. When you praise a man, he will be motivated and encouraged to be better. Remember, at his core, he wants to please you and be the one you need.

2. Look inward and examine your own life. Are you cultivating your mind, heart, and spirit? Do you read substantive works, develop your individuality, and form opinions? Do you peer at the world through a prism of vibrancy and color? Do you choose to be joyous and rise above the provocations of the

small stuff? Do you find the hidden within the revealed and the miraculous within the natural? Are you in touch with the divine mystery that surrounds you?

3. Speak to other women and hear the way they find your husband masculine and sexy—there will be some who do. Whenever a wife hears another woman talk about her husband in this way, interest is renewed and passion kindled.

4. Acknowledge to yourself that men find you attractive. Don't court it purposefully, but realize you're a mysterious, sexual woman. Simply, be aware of male attention.

5. Allow people's attention to feed your confidence. You're desirable, and you know it. Absorb encompassing sexual energy and bring it home to your husband. Be aware of your environment.

6. Mention to your husband the attention strangers have given you. Be casual about it. Your intent is to get him to notice you in a different light, not to arouse unhealthy jealousy. You have to always be sensitive to how you affect his confidence and his trust in you by what you say. It should be understood as a delicate, sexy dance between you—he should know and understand that you are giving him something to help him desire you more, something to make him feel better about the fact that you are his. It should never be done to trip him up or to diminish his self-worth. If you're doing that, you're doing it wrong, and you should stop and try something else instead.

7. Lead a full life. Don't morph into your husband or have the marriage totally usurp your identity. Indulge hobbies, contribute to your community, take online classes, volunteer for important organizations. You're a wife. But you're also a person. Safeguard your individuality.

8. As much as you can afford it, purchase new sexy underwear and bras to wear for your husband. Twice a month would be perfect if you can do it. In the morning, as you get dressed, or at night when you go to sleep, model it for him. Simply say, "Oh, I got this yesterday, how does it look?"

9. Take erotic pictures of yourself that only your husband will see. Safely send them to him or leave them for him to find. If you can get a professional female photographer to take the pictures, do it. Have fun with it!

10. Remain mysterious even at home. Don't let your husband see you change your clothes. If you do, dim the lights so he only sees your outline, making him want to see more. Wear sexy undergarments—be the mistress.

11. Don't go out of your way to answer your cell phone every time he calls or texts. Your husband doesn't need to reach you every single minute. You can afford to be a little inaccessible sometimes. The anticipation will make him long for you and want you even more. This isn't to say that you should ignore him. It just means that you don't have to be a slave to his attentions. If you love him, you will naturally want to get back to him immediately, but that can have the opposite effect to the one you intend. Do your thing. Look after your work and interests, and don't drop everything just because he's texting you. Your work is also important. Remember, independence is sexy too.

12. Dress differently for your husband than you do for other men. Set aside certain outfits that you only wear for him. Make him feel special.

13. Kiss your husband at every available opportunity. Soften him up by showing affection, get him to talk about his emotions, and listen. Show him that real strength and courage is letting go of the fear of being tender.

14. Light candles around the house to bring a feminine glow to the home. It will soften the mood and foster romance.

15. Read an erotic novel before bed. Show your husband you're thinking about sex. Tell him your dreams about sex, even if a stranger makes a guest appearance. If he starts to get angry, make sure he knows there is nothing to worry about. When you dream about sex with someone else, it doesn't mean that you ever want to cheat. It can often be your desire for an aspect of your partner that is being revealed by the subconscious in the dream. It's an opportunity to discover something about your partner sexually. And your partner will react better if you tell him that you want to hear about his dreams too.

16. Become his fantasy—a seductive siren. We've talked about how men are often tired of always having to play the role of provider—to be responsible and in control. What he wants from his lover is to experience release. Robert Greene in *The Art of Seduction* explains: "The Siren is the ultimate male fantasy figure because she offers a total release from the limitations of his life. In her presence, which is always heightened and sexually charged, the male feels transported to a world of pure pleasure. She is dangerous, and In pursuing her energetically the man can lose control over himself, something he yearns to do. The Siren is a mirage; she lures men by cultivating a particular appearance and manner. In a world where women are often too timid to project such an image, learn to take control of the male libido by embodying his fantasy."[1] To know what your partner wants, you will need to ask him. Communication is key, as is radical honesty. Get to know the dark impulses and tap into them. Become the fantasy.

Channeling Your Masculinity

Like an apple tree among the trees of the forest is my beloved among the young men. I delight to sit in his shade, and his fruit is sweet to my taste.

SONG OF SOLOMON

Women want to be desired, and a man wants to be the only one who can feed her hunger. Here are some ways a man can cultivate sexual tension with his wife.

1. Tell your wife how beautiful she is and how much you admire everything she does. Tell her she's a superwoman for balancing all the many aspects of her life. Praise her, encourage her, and recharge her when she is drained by all the many things she has to do every day. Focus on the positive, and she will melt in your arms.

2. Look inward and examine your own life. What could you be doing better? Do you show enough appreciation to your wife? Do you say thank you even for the little things she does? Are you doing everything you can for her or are you

consumed with yourself and your own interests? Do you try
to make life better for her or harder? Be honest with yourself
no matter how difficult, and make changes. She will notice
and love you more for it. If passion is moribund in your
marriage, go to a bar with your wife and let her sit separate
from you. Watch what happens next. Pretend you don't know
her. This will incite a sprinkling of jealousy and remind you of
how sexy your wife is.

3. Ask your wife to tell you what kind of men are attracted to
   her. Don't belittle the men, but merely tell her, "Of course
   he'd be attracted to you. Look at how beautiful you are."
   Really let her know how sexy you think she is.

4. Be interested in her. Always be trying to discover new things
   about your wife. Don't just ask her about her day—and
   definitely don't ignore her. Find out details. Ask her about
   her feelings, her perspectives. Show that she's a compelling,
   interesting woman. Be curious and delve into the infinite
   mystery that is your wife.

5. When making love to your wife and it feels like the erotic
   energies are burning low, imagine her with a stranger. Focus
   the fantasy on your wife and her desirability.

6. If your marriage is emotionally strong and your ego can
   handle it, ask her to tell you who she thinks is attractive
   (wives, don't let this be someone close to you—that could
   create conflict). Allow this to remind you of her existence as
   a sexual being—to once again see her desire. In turn you will
   desire her more. When you're tempted to think about other
   women, think of your wife with this other man. Use this to
   counterbalance your temptations. Let her sexuality draw your
   mind back to her.

7. Build anticipation by always keeping your wife on the edge about when you're going to have sex. Be passionate and spontaneous. Some days, get dressed in your suit and tie only to rip it off a few moments later just when she thinks you went out to the car to leave.

8. Pay attention to her. Watch your wife as she moves around the house; take in her femininity, and let it fuel your imagination.

9. When making love, be sure your wife has an orgasm before you do. Pleasure her first.

10. Seduce your wife. At least once a week, give her a long sensual massage. Do it when she's tired from a long day of work. She might not want to, but she'll start to relax, and passion will stir. It's getting her into the mood that's erotic.

11. Take good care of your wife. If she's not feeling well, make her breakfast in bed, take care of the children, fix dinner and serve it with a rose. Become the radiant knight in shining armor who protects and cares for her.

12. Be active. Women aren't turned on by slothful men. Be motivated and energetic. Don't be a couch potato.

13. Exercise together. She'll appreciate your effort to stay fit and she'll get to see you sweat.

14. Take charge in the bedroom. This doesn't have to happen all the time, but women want to be swept off their feet at least some of the time. When she's receptive, grab your wife and make love to her—right there on the living room floor, on the kitchen table, wherever. Taking charge with strong masculine energy attracts her feminine energy, and when they come together, it's explosive.

15. Talk to your wife about your anxieties, vulnerabilities, and fears. Let her inside of your soul. Don't worry about not appearing macho. She wants to see this part of you. Allow yourself to open up even if you're afraid of getting hurt. Invite her into your deepest, most intimate spaces.

Parents Are Still Lovers

Children always assume the sexual lives of their parents come to a grinding halt at their conception.

ALAN BENNETT

O ne of romance's most fatal foes can be a beloved child. When a baby comes into the world, everything changes. Those hours you once spent in meaningful conversation and passionate lovemaking suddenly transform into changing diapers, rocking a crying baby late into the night, and cleaning spit-up from your clothes. Research shows that sexual intercourse drops by more than 40 percent in the year following the birth of a child.[1] Too often when we become parents, we think our life as lovers is over. We're tired, distracted, and consumed with the needs of a new human being entrusted to our care. Who has time for sex—the kids come first.

This is the wrong way to think about it. It's unhealthy both for parents and their children. Instead of love for children disrupting the love between a husband and wife, the parents' love for each other should be the spring that flows over to the children. Parents need to show their children love in action, not just love in theory. The former is taught by loving your children; the latter is shown by loving your spouse. When you love your kids, they experience love, but when you love your spouse, they are seeing love modeled before them. This is the best gift you can give your children—showing them the love between a husband and wife. If they don't have that example in their lives, they won't know the security of that love and they won't learn how to passionately love someone when they're older.

When parents model love in front of their children, they are raising children to be loving themselves. One of the best ways to bring about a sensual revolution in our society is to raise children who value intimacy and desire, horizontal exploration and vertical renewal, love and passion. By providing them healthy examples, they will mimic what they see. Parents also need to actively teach them how to be great lovers by having them spend time listening and engaging in meaningful conversation, putting away technology and enjoying nature, serving others instead of always having their needs and wants catered to, and nourishing their souls with spiritual instruction.

Recharging your sex life after childbirth is important to maintain a vibrant, loving relationship that will be a testimony to your children of the sustainability of love in long-term monogamous relationships. Here are some tips to keep passion alive after beloved little ones come into your life.

1. Keep some spaces sacred. Be aware that if you allow your children to always sleep in your bedroom, it can begin to erode the excitement and privilege of this space—the inner sanctum of your marriage. It is natural for children to reach out for their parents in the dark, but it is healthier and better for the child if they learn to feel safe and secure in their own beds. Make sure they understand and respect that this is your personal space, and that it can only happen occasionally. Take them back to their rooms, and make sure they come to understand.

2. Never talk about children and household issues during lovemaking. This seems obvious but needs to be said. Focus your mind on your spouse, not on the kids.

3. Plan for a honeymoon getaway at least two times a year. It doesn't have to be expensive. Just make arrangements for relatives to keep the kids, and the two of you go off and enjoy each other in a new setting—make it a kind of ongoing honeymoon. This is not a waste of money—it is a wise investment in your marriage.

4. Set aside a couple-only night at least once a week. It can be a date or just time you spend together—not watching television or a movie, but talking, emotionally connecting, and engaging in vertical discovery.

5. Spend at least fifteen minutes every day not talking about the children. Have real, intimate conversation about each other without the distractions of routine and domestic responsibilities. You're adults. You need this. You need to be filled.

6. Get physical with each other. Not just sex, but hugging, kissing, snuggling. When you get home from work, hug each other in a long sensual embrace. Children need to see their parents touching, and you need to be touched!

7. Get some help around the house. If you can manage it, get help with housework and childcare so you're not so exhausted when your spouse comes home. This isn't neglecting your duties; it's investing in your marriage, which is foundational to everything else.

8. Declare family time over at 9 p.m. every night. Spend time with the family from 6 to 9 p.m., eating, bathing, reading, helping with homework, and talking about whatever interests your kids. When the clock hits 9 p.m., mom and dad time begins, and they're not to be disturbed. Little children are in bed, and teenagers keep to themselves. This protects the intimacy of the parents and gives them space to relax from the long day and, hopefully, to make love.

Practicing Passionate Connectedness

*The source of all life and knowledge is in man and woman, and
the source of all living is in the interchange and the meeting and
mingling of these two: man-life and woman-life, man-knowledge
and woman-knowledge, man-being and woman-being.*

D. H. LAWRENCE

C entral to rediscovering the lost art of intimacy is the synthesis of
love and desire, passion and practicality, friends and lovers. This
is how passionate connectedness is created. Here are some tips on
how this is accomplished.

1. Practice conversational intimacy. Keep all talk about your sex
   life in the bedroom between the two of you. That's where
   it belongs. Don't discuss your sex life with anyone else. A
   couple's problems and issues are their problems (or their
   counselor's or therapist's problems, where applicable). Too
   many people discuss intimate aspects of their marriages
   with friends. This is a betrayal of your intimate relationship.
   Instead, maintain intimacy through exclusivity. Treat your
   relationship as sacred.

2. Practice mental fidelity. If you allow yourself to become excited by other people, your attraction to your spouse and your erotic dependence on him will be lessened. When people watch porn, flirt with others, or think about someone else while making love to their spouse, they are directing their primary sex organ—the brain—outside their marriage. This diminishes the focus that's needed for true erotic intensity within a relationship. Instead of indulging these thoughts, see them as an opportunity to focus your sexual energy back into your relationship.

3. Recognize the power of natural sexual attraction between the masculine and feminine. Men, embrace your full masculinity. Women, express your femininity unapologetically. Eroticism is rooted in the attraction of the polar opposites. In heterosexual relationships, a man is drawn to a woman's powerful feminine nature because it completes him, fulfills him, and satisfies his hunger like nothing else. The same is true for a woman. A man's masculine presence inflames her desire, and the erotic tension that is created is explosive.

4. Fantasize about your spouse in erotic situations. Create a sense of newness about them by mentally placing them in novel situations. Be your own movie director and let your imagination roam. Be creative.

5. Write love letters and poetry to one another. Leave love notes around the house, under pillows, in books, on the dashboard of the car.

6. Never put yourself in situations where the small embers of attraction to someone else will catch fire. Don't laugh off all those little erotic attractions you feel. These will either have to be suppressed or they'll naturally grow. Neither is good

for a marriage. If you're flirting with other people, you're
diluting erotic desire for your spouse. This is especially true
with online interaction. Don't spend your time on your phone
or computer when you should be focusing on your spouse.
If you're always holding a screen up to your face, you're
not paying attention to your spouse. This creates unhealthy
jealousies. The next thing you know, your spouse is checking
your computer histories, stalking you on social media, trying
to find any hint of infidelity. Pamela's father once told her that
suspicion within a relationship is self-fulfilling. He said that "if
you look hard enough for something, you will find it." This
can ruin a relationship. So, put down the gadgets, stop flirting
with others, and put your erotic energy into your spouse.

7. It's not necessary to be open about everything. Maintain
some privacy zones. Don't bring up past lovers to your
spouse. Even if your spouse wants to talk about it, don't. If
you do, they will inevitably feel that you're comparing them
in some way. It's time to bury the ghosts of the past and
leave them buried.

8. Remember the power of missionary. The missionary position
is often scorned as boring, but this is missing the importance
of sensual connection. It takes commitment—it's full-body
contact, face to face, eyes looking deeply into the eyes of
another. This is the most intimate two people can get. This
is the best way to practice vertical exploration—you can
look into your partner's soul, engage their mind, and explore
their spirit. You breathe in each other, kiss, touch, talk. When
making love, *look* at each other. Don't just have sex and get
it over with. Build intimacy through physical connection.

9. For men: Make a conscious decision to derive erotic interest
exclusively from your wife. Those casual exchanges with a

stranger can, in fact, be tiny erotic encounters. It might seem totally innocent, but if you're honest with yourself you'll acknowledge that's not completely true. Everyone needs to have his or her erotic mind fed. When you spread your attentions all around, you're reducing the intensity in your marriage. Learn to fix your erotic attention only on your wife. Stare at her when she bends down and look for the outline of her undergarments. See the sensual woman in your wife. Steal flirtatious moments during the day to say something affectionate. Watch her interactions with other men and be reminded of her intrinsic attractiveness. They see her womanhood. Noticing this helps you see her through the eyes of another to whom she is novel and new. By keeping your erotic attention focused on your wife, you're feeding your erotic attraction to her.

10. For women: Make a conscious decision to derive erotic interest exclusively from your husband. Today, women are just as open to flirting with strangers as men. Many women feel they are not getting the kind of attention they really want in their relationship at home, so they look outside for what they need. Women, like men, get a great deal of erotic pleasure from other people through casual conversation. But, there are consequences to this. Flirting with other men causes a diminishment of primary attraction to your husband. You might still love him, but you just don't desire him as much. Instead of flirting, tell your husband about the men who show you attention—not to create artificial jealousy but to start an erotic conversation that captures the fullness of your sexuality and your everyday erotic experiences. Bring them into your marriage.

11. Remember that unavailability is a prime condition of desire, and use the times when you are apart to build your attraction. If one of you has to travel, send each other erotic notes, talk on the phone, and generally work yourselves into a frenzy that you will consummate when you are reunited. You can even do this during the workday, so long as you don't neglect your responsibilities.

12. Don't treat your wife like a maid, mother, homemaker, and caretaker or even a fellow provider. When the practical overshadows the erotic, your wife doesn't feel like a woman anymore. A husband needs to bring out his wife's desire. Jewish values have a lot to say on this. One is that a woman should be pleasured *before* her husband. Seeing his wife give herself over to wild erotic abandon creates desire in a husband too. It's a win-win.

13. Don't treat your husband like nothing more than a workhorse provider. Men, like women, want to be valued for more than just the paycheck. Most men are very happy to provide for their families, but a man wants to feel like more than a cash machine and a handyman. He needs to feel valued for who he is and not just for what he can do. Women today are nearly equal financial providers for the family. So they know that while career is very important, we still all want to be appreciated for our being as much as for our doing.

14. Realize that the little things are not little. We tend to think that as long as spouses are not committing technical infidelity or engaging in extremely compromising behavior, then anything goes. But it's a choice you're making: where are you going to invest your erotic energy? Where you invest is where you will see returns.

15. Practice romance. Do things for each other that simply build up desirability. Give each other little gifts. When you're shopping, stop and give each other a hug and kiss. Show affection, touch, look at one another. Flirt. Hold hands. Give each other compliments and never say anything demeaning. Take walks together. Sit outside and look at the stars while you listen to music. Light candles and sit cross-legged on the bed and talk. Read erotic literature to one another. Take a long bath together. Whatever you can think of—make time for romance.

16. Tell each other thank you. Show appreciation for everything the other does. Look for ways to serve one another—and always show how thankful you are. Service and appreciation fuel love.

17. Laugh together. Laughter is sexy. It heals, relieves stress, lightens the heart, and drives away fear. Fyodor Dostoyevsky once said, "If you wish to glimpse inside a human soul and get to know a man, don't bother analyzing his ways of being silent, of talking, of weeping, of seeing how much he is moved by noble ideas; you will get better results if you just watch him laugh. If he laughs well, he's a good man." One could also say when a couple laughs well together, their relationship is good.

18. Don't be lazy! Keeping love and passion alive isn't easy. It takes work. Just because you're wearing a ring doesn't mean you can check out. Love should be forever, but it doesn't last on sheer inertia. You have to keep pushing, trying, and striving. Trust us, it's worth it.

CONCLUSION

The stakes are too high for us to ignore our flat-lining sex lives. If we don't give our relationships the care and attention they need, our society will only descend further into loneliness and anxiety. It should be a no-brainer—who doesn't want to have more and better sex? Who doesn't want to have a more passionate life? But as we have shown, the modern, post–sexual revolution era has warped our concepts of sex and sexuality.

We are proposing a sensual revolution, a rediscovery of intimacy, that encourages and ennobles human relationships, that gets us from looking up from the glowing screens of our smart phones to the people around us, most especially the people we love the most. This is one reason the Jewish Bible started the ritual of the Sabbath, of keeping one day per week holy from the corrosive effects of technology. The benefits of reducing our overuse of technology—especially the Internet—are far reaching, and they include better human connections and spiritual renewal. But one of the greatest rewards is happier, more sensual relationships.

We hope this book has explained the problem and offered real, work-able solutions that can be practiced by men and women in all kinds of relationships—married and not married. We hope our intervention—the shared insights of a *Playboy* model and a Rabbi—can begin to address the sexual confusion of the modern mind. A happier, more fulfilling, more intimate future is ahead, and won't we all have fun getting there together?

ENDNOTES

Preface by Pamela Anderson

1 Nin, Anaïs. *The Diary of Anaïs Nin*. Boston, Houghton Mifflin Harcourt, 1969.
2 Ibid.
3 Ibid.

Chapter 1: The Art of Intimacy

1 Nin, Anaïs. *Delta of Venus*. London, Penguin Books, 2007.

Chapter 2: Our Deep Need

1 Larkin, Philip. "Talking In Bed." All Poetry, https://allpoetry.com/Talking-In-Bed.

Chapter 3: A Sexual Famine

1 Fromm, Erich. *The Art of Loving*. New York, Continuum, 2008.
2 Nin, Anaïs. *Delta of Venus*. London, Penguin Books, 2007.
3 Tshemese, Amanda. "Lack of Sexual Intimacy Linked to Depression in Women: Study." *SABC News*, 4 March 2015, www.sabc.co.za/news/a/06d0408047857038a0fee642d945d4b0/Lack-of-sexual-intimacy-linked-to-depression-in-women:-Study-20150304.
4 Ibid.
5 "Six out of 10 Couples 'Unhappy in Their Relationship'." *Daily Mail Online*, Associated Newspapers, 31 May 2010, www.dailymail.co.uk/news/article-1282851/Six-10-couples-unhappy-relationship.html.
6 Ibid.
7 Ibid.
8 Ibid.
9 "May your fountain be blessed, and may you rejoice in the wife of your youth. A loving doe, a graceful deer—may her breasts satisfy you always, may you ever be intoxicated with her love." Proverbs 5:18–19. *The Holy Bible, New International Version*. Grand Rapids, MI, Zondervan, 1984.
10 Deveny, Kathleen. "We're Not in the Mood." *Newsweek*, 13 March 2010, www.newsweek.com/were-not-mood-138387.

11 "Relationships in America Survey." *Introduction | Relationships in America*, The Austin Institute for the Study of Family and Culture, 2014, relationshipsinamerica.com/.

12 Laumann, Edward O. *The Social Organization of Sexuality: Sexual Practices in the United States.* Chicago, University of Chicago Press, 2002. Print.

13 Donnelly, Denise A. "Sexually Inactive Marriages." *Journal of Sex Research* 30.2 (1993): 171–79. www.tandfonline.com/doi/abs/10.1080/00224499309551698?src=recsys.

14 "Relationships in America Survey."

15 Twenge, Jean M., et al. "Declines in Sexual Frequency among American Adults, 1989–2014." *Archives of Sexual Behavior*, June 2017, doi:10.1007/s10508-017-0953-1.

16 Ibid.

17 "The Decline of Marriage and Rise of New Families." *Pew Research Center's Social & Demographic Trends Project*, 17 November 2010, www.pewsocialtrends .org/2010/11/18/the-decline-of-marriage-and-rise-of-new-families/.

18 Twenge, "Declines in Sexual Frequency among American Adults, 1989–2014."

19 Ibid.

20 Ibid.

21 DePaulo, Bella. "Marriage and Happiness: 18 Long-Term Studies." *Psychology Today*, Sussex Publishers, 15 March 2013, www.psychologytoday.com/ blog/living-single/201303/marriage-and-happiness-18-long-term-studies.

22 "World Happiness Report 2017." *World Happiness Report*, worldhappiness.report/ed/2017/.

23 Twenge, Jean M., et al. "More Happiness for Young People and Less for Mature Adults." *Social Psychological and Personality Science* 7 (2016): 131–41. doi:10.1177/1948550615602933.

24 "Too Much Texting Can Disconnect Couples, Research Finds." *Brigham Young University*, 26 May 2016, news.byu.edu/news/too-much-texting-can-disconnect-couples-research-finds.

25 "I have come into my garden, my sister, my bride; I have gathered my myrrh with my spice. I have eaten my honeycomb and my honey; I have drunk my wine and my milk." Song of Solomon 5:1. *The Holy Bible, New International Version*. Grand Rapids, MI, Zondervan, 1984.

26 Livingston, Gretchen, and Andrea Caumont. "5 Facts on Love and Marriage in America." *Pew Research Center*, 13 February 2017, www.pewresearch.org/fact-tank/2017/02/13/ 5-facts-about-love-and-marriage/.

27 Ibid.

28 Ibid.

29 Ibid.

Chapter 4: Failure of the Sexual Revolution

1 Genesis 2:24. *King James Bible*. Nashville, TN, Holman Bible Publishers, 1973.

2 Song of Solomon 4:3–7. *The Holy Bible, New International Version*. Grand Rapids, MI, Zondervan, 1984.

3 Fromm, Erich. *The Art of Loving*. New York, Continuum, 2008.

4 Ibid.

5 Oz, Mehmet. "The New Loneliness." *The Huffington Post*, TheHuffingtonPost.com, 12 September 2016, www.huffingtonpost.com/dr-mehmet-oz/the-new-loneliness _b_11966516.html.

6 Mcpherson, Miller, et al. "Social Isolation in America: Changes in Core Discussion
   Networks over Two Decades." *American Sociological Review* 71 (2006): 353–75.
   doi:10.1177/000312240807300610.

7 Entis, Laura. "Chronic Loneliness Is a Modern-Day Epidemic." *Fortune.com*, 22 June 2016,
   fortune.com/2016/06/22/loneliness-is-a-modern-day-epidemic/.

8 Tanizaki, Jun'ichiro. *The Key*. London, Vintage, 2004.

9 Warren, Rossalyn. "42 of the Best, Worst, and Weirdest Messages Ever Sent on Tinder."
   BuzzFeed, www.buzzfeed.com/rossalynwarren/best-worst-and-weirdest-messages
   -tinder?utm_term=.xu2EqDP6Q#.jjrZKEX24.

10 McKernan, Bethan. "20 of the Best Worst Messages Ever
   Sent on Tinder." *Indy100*, 20 June 2015, www.indy100.com/
   article/20-of-the-best-worst-messages-ever-sent-on-tinder--ZJMpxicobe.

11 Warren, "42 of the Best, Worst, and Weirdest Messages Ever Sent on Tinder."

Chapter 5: Is Porn for Losers?

1 Kahlo, Frida, and Martha Zamora. *The Letters of Frida Kahlo: Cartas Apasionadas*. San Francisco,
   Chronicle Books, 1995.

2 American Academy of Matrimonial Lawyers. "Is the Internet Bad for Your Marriage? Online
   Affairs, Pornographic Sites Playing Greater Role in Divorces." *PR Newswire: News Distribution,
   Targeting and Monitoring*, 13 November 2002, www.prnewswire.com/news-releases/is-the
   -Internet-bad-for-your-marriage-online-affairs-pornographic-sites-playing-greater-role-in
   -divorces-76826727.html.

3 Reisman, Judith, Jeffrey Sanitover, Mary Anne Layden, and James B. Weaver. "Hearing
   on the Brain Science Behind Pornography Addiction and the Effects of Addiction on
   Families and Communities." Hearing to the U.S. Senate Committee on Commerce,
   Science, and Transportation. November 18, 2004. http://www.drjudithreisman.com/
   archives/2011/06/2004_testimony.html.

4 Ibid.

5 Zillmann, Dolf, and Jennings Bryant. "Pornography's Impact on Sexual Satisfaction." *Journal
   of Applied Social Psychology*, Blackwell Publishing Ltd, 31 April 1988. onlinelibrary.wiley.com/
   doi/10.1111/j.1559-1816.1988.tb00027.x/abstract.

6 Ibid.

7 Zillmann, Dolf. "The Effects of Prolonged Consumption of Pornography." In: Zillmann, Dolf,
   and Jennings Bryant, editors. *Pornography: Research Advances and Policy Considerations*. Hillsdale,
   NJ, Lawrence Erlbaum, 1989.

8 Gwinn, Andrea Marlea, et al. "Pornography, Relationship Alternatives, and Intimate
   Extradyadic Behavior." *Social Psychological and Personality Science* 4 (2013): 699–704.
   doi:10.1177/1948550613480821.

9 Maddox, Amanda M., et al. "Viewing Sexually-Explicit Materials Alone or Together:
   Associations with Relationship Quality." *Archives of Sexual Behavior* 40 (2009): 441–48.
   doi:10.1007/s10508-009-9585-4.

10 Ibid.

11 Lambert, Nathaniel M., et al. "A Love That Doesn't Last: Pornography Consumption and
   Weakened Commitment to One's Romantic Partner." *Journal of Social and Clinical Psychology* 31
   (2012): 410–38. doi:10.1521/jscp.2012.31.4.410.

12 Kenrick, Douglas T., et al. "Influence of Popular Erotica on Judgments of
    Strangers and Mates." *Journal of Experimental Social Psychology* 25 (1989): 159–67.
    doi:10.1016/0022-1031(89)90010-3.

13 Ibid.

14 Reisman, "Hearing on the Brain Science Behind Pornography Addiction and the Effects of
    Addiction on Families and Communities."

15 Park, Brian, et al. "Is Internet Pornography Causing Sexual Dysfunctions? A Review with
    Clinical Reports." *Behavioral Sciences* 6 (2016): E17. doi:10.3390/bs6030017.

16 Ibid.

17 Ibid.

18 Pratt, Russ. "The 'Porn Genie' Is out of the Bottle: Understanding and Responding to the
    Impact of Pornography on Young People." *Australian Psychological Society*, 14 April 2015, www
    .psychology.org.au/inpsych/2015/april/pratt/.

19 Ibid.

20 Hald, Gert Martin, et al. "Pornography and Attitudes Supporting Violence against Women:
    Revisiting the Relationship in Nonexperimental Studies." *Aggressive Behavior* 36 (2010): 14–20.
    doi:10.1002/ab.20328.

21 Gholipour, Bahar. "Teen Anal Sex Study: 6 Unexpected Findings." *LiveScience*, Purch, 13 August
    2014, www.livescience.com/47352-teen-anal-sex-unexpected-findings.html.

22 Ibid.

23 Ibid.

24 Ibid.

25 Ibid.

26 Twenge, Jean M., et al. "Sexual Inactivity During Young Adulthood Is More Common
    Among U.S. Millennials and IGen: Age, Period, and Cohort Effects on Having
    No Sexual Partners After Age 18." *Archives of Sexual Behavior* 46 (2016): 433–40.
    doi:10.1007/s10508-016-0798-z.

27 Bahrampour, Tara. "'There Isn't Really Anything Magical about It': Why More Millennials Are
    Avoiding Sex." *The Washington Post*, WP Company, 2 August 2016, www.washingtonpost
    .com/local/social-issues/there-isnt-really-anything-magical-about-it-why-more-millennials
    -are-putting-off-sex/2016/08/02/e7b73d6e-37f4-11e6-8f7c-d4c723a2becb_story
    .html?utm_term.

28 Ibid.

29 Braun-Courville, Debra K., and Mary Rojas. "Exposure to Sexually Explicit Web Sites and
    Adolescent Sexual Attitudes and Behaviors." *Journal of Adolescent Health* 45 (2009): 156–62.
    doi:10.1016/j.jadohealth.2008.12.004.

Chapter 7: Too Much of a Good Thing

1 *Marvin Miller v. State of California*. Holding: "Obscene materials are defined as those that the
   average person, applying contemporary community standards, find, taken as a whole, appeal
   to the prurient interest; that depict or describe, in a patently offensive way, sexual conduct or
   excretory functions specifically defined by applicable state law; and that the work, taken as a
   whole, lack serious literary, artistic, political, or scientific value."

2   Sales, Nancy Jo. "Tinder and the Dawn of the 'Dating Apocalypse.'" *Vanity Fair*, 15 September 2016, www.vanityfair.com/culture/2015/08/tinder-hookup-culture-end-of-dating.

3   Ibid.

4   Ibid.

5   Ibid.

6   Ibid.

7   Ibid.

8   Ibid.

9   Fromm, Erich. *The Art of Loving*. New York, Continuum, 2008.

10 Ibid.

11 Ibid.

12 Ross, Carolyn. "Overexposed and Under-Prepared: The Effects of Early Exposure to Sexual Content." *Psychology Today*, Sussex Publishers, 13 August 2012, www.psychologytoday.com/blog/real-healing/201208/overexposed-and-under-prepared-the-effects-early-exposure-sexual-content.

13 Twenge, Jean M., et al. "Changes in American Adults' Sexual Behavior and Attitudes, 1972–2012." *Archives of Sexual Behavior* 44 (2015): 2273–85. doi:10.1007/s10508-015-0540-2.

14 Ibid.

15 Ibid.

16 "Report of the APA Task Force on the Sexualization of Girls." *American Psychological Association*, www.apa.org/pi/women/programs/girls/report.aspx.

17 Ibid.

18 Ibid.

19 Ibid.

20 Ibid.

21 St. John, Warren. "In an Oversexed Age, More Guys Take a Pill." *The New York Times*, 14 December 2003, www.nytimes.com/2003/12/14/style/in-an-oversexed-age-more-guys-take-a-pill.html.

22 Ibid.

23 Ibid.

24 Ibid.

25 Ibid.

26 Ibid.

27 Ibid.

28 Ibid.

29 Ibid.

30 Twenge, "Changes in American Adults' Sexual Behavior and Attitudes, 1972–2012."

31 Ibid.

32 Ibid.

33 Twenge, Jean M., et al. "Sexual Inactivity During Young Adulthood Is More Common Among U.S. Millennials and IGen: Age, Period, and Cohort Effects on Having No Sexual Partners After Age 18." *Archives of Sexual Behavior* 46 (2016): 433–40. doi:10.1007/s10508-016-0798-z.

34 Ibid.

35 "Hookup Culture Leaves Students Wanting." *Harvard News*, www.thecrimson.com/article/2012/3/27/sex-week-hookups/.

36 Ibid.
37 Ibid.
38 Ibid.
39 Ibid.
40 Ibid.
41 Ibid.
42 NPR. "'Girls & Sex' and the Importance of Talking to Young Women About Pleasure." *Fresh Air*, NPR, 29 March 2016, www.npr.org/sections/health-shots/2016/03/29/472211301/girls -sex-and-the-importance-of-talking-to-young-women-about-pleasure.
43 Ibid.
44 Ibid.
45 Ibid.

Chapter 8: Becoming Sexual Experts

1 Fromm, Erich. *The Art of Loving*. New York, Continuum, 2008.
2 Langton, Rae. *Sexual Solipsism: Philosophical Essays on Pornography and Objectification*. Oxford, Oxford University Press, 2009.

Chapter 9: Goal-Oriented Sex

1 Allahdadi, Kyan J., et al. "Female Sexual Dysfunction: Therapeutic Options and Experimental Challenges." *Cardiovascular & Hematological Agents in Medicinal Chemistry*, U.S. National Library of Medicine, October 2009, www.ncbi.nlm.nih.gov/pmc/articles/PMC3008577/.
2 Howard, Jacqueline. "Who Orgasms Most and Least, and Why." *CNN*, Cable News Network, 10 March 2017, www.cnn.com/2017/03/10/health/orgasm-frequency-sex-explainer -study/index.html.
3 Ibid.

Chapter 11: Captured by Desire

1 Isaiah 54:5, *Holy Bible, New International Version*, NIV® Copyright ©1973, 1978, 1984, 2011 by Biblica, Inc.® Used by permission. All rights reserved worldwide.
2 Hosea 2:19–20, *Holy Bible, New International Version*.
3 Goble, Paul. *Love Flute*. New York, Aladdin Paperbacks, 1997.
4 Ibid.
5 Ibid.
6 Bergner, Daniel. "What Do Women Want?" *The New York Times*, 24 January 2009, www.nytimes .com/2009/01/25/magazine/25desire-t.html.
7 Ibid.
8 Ibid.
9 Ibid.
10 Ibid.
11 Ibid.
12 Ibid.

13 Ibid.
14 Ibid.
15 Ibid.
16 Ibid.
17 Ibid.
18 Ibid.

Chapter 12: Erotic Fantasy

1   "Wives: Want to Be Ravished?" *The Marriage Bed*, 18 May 2015, site.themarriagebed.com/
    surveys/wives-want-to-be-ravished/.
2   Elton, Catherine. "Learning to Lust." *Psychology Today*, Sussex Publishers, 1 May 2010, www
    .psychologytoday.com/articles/201005/learning-lust.
3   Bergner, Daniel. "What Do Women Want?" *The New York Times*, 24 January 2009, www.nytimes
    .com/2009/01/25/magazine/25desire-t.html.
4   Ibid.
5   Ibid.
6   Ibid.
7   Ibid.

Chapter 13: Passionate Connectedness

1   Fanthorpe, Ursula A., and Carol Ann Duffy. "Atlas." *New and Collected Poems*. London,
    Enitharmon Press, 2010.
2   Estés, Clarissa Pinkola. *Women Who Run with the Wolves: Myths and Stories of the Wild Woman
    Archetype* (Kindle Locations 2287-2290). Kindle Edition.
3   Fahs, Breanne. *Performing Sex: The Making and Unmaking of Women's Erotic Lives*. Albany, State
    University of New York Press, 2011.
4   Ibid.
5   Ibid.
6   Ibid.
7   "Women More Likely than Men to Initiate Divorces, but Not Non-Marital Breakups."
    ScienceDaily, 22 August 2017, www.sciencedaily.com/releases/2015/08/150822154900
    .htm.
8   Ibid.
9   Laughlin, James. "O Best of All Nights, Return and Return Again," from *Poems New and Selected*.
    Copyright © 1996 by James Laughlin. Reprinted with the permission of New Directions
    Publishing Corporation.
10 Gibran, Kahlil. *The Complete Works of Kahlil Gibran*. New Delhi, Published by Indiana Pub.
    House for Cross Land Books, 2008.

Chapter 14: Give a Woman What She Wants

1   Adams, Bryan. "Have You Ever Really Loved a Woman?" *18 til I Die*, A&M, 1995.

2 Estés, Clarissa Pinkola. *Women Who Run with the Wolves: Myths and Stories of the Wild Woman Archetype* (Kindle Locations 2287-2290). Kindle Edition.
3 Ibid.
4 Ibid.

Chapter 15: Needing To Be Needed

1 Napoleon, and Henry Foljambe Hall. *Napoleon's Letters to Josephine, 1796–1812. For the First Time Collected and Translated, with Notes from Contemporary Sources, by H.F. Hall*. J.M. Dent & Co., 1901.
2 Ibid.
3 Ibid.
4 Weber, Jill P. "What Do Men Need From Women? 5 Insights." *Psychology Today*, Sussex Publishers, 30 October 2014, www.psychologytoday.com/blog/having-sex-wanting-intimacy/201410/what-do-men-need-women-5-insights.
5 Liedloff, Jean. *The Continuum Concept: In Search of Happiness*. Cambridge, MA, De Capo Press, 1975.
6 Ibid.
7 Jaffe, Eric. "What Do Men Really Want?" *Psychology Today*, Sussex Publishers, 13 March 2012, www.psychologytoday.com/articles/201203/what-do-men-really-want.
8 Ibid.
9 Gray, John. *Men Are from Mars, Women Are from Venus: Practical Guide for Improving Communication* (Kindle Locations 859-864). HarperCollins. Kindle Edition.
10 Neruda, Pablo, and Donald D. Walsh. "Your Laughter." *Love Poems*. New York, New Directions Book, 2008.
11 Estés, Clarissa Pinkola. *Women Who Run with the Wolves: Myths and Stories of the Wild Woman Archetype* (Kindle Locations 2287-2290). Kindle Edition.
12 Whitman, Walt, and Francis Murphy. "A Glimpse." *The Complete Poems Walt Whitman*. Harmondsworth, Penguin Education, 1975.

Chapter 16: Masculine Duality

1 Estés, Clarissa Pinkola. *Women Who Run with the Wolves: Myths and Stories of the Wild Woman Archetype* (Kindle Locations 2287-2290). Kindle Edition.
2 Hozier, Andrew, and Sallay-Matu Garnett. "Someone New." Sony/ATV Music Publishing LLC.
3 Job 34:4, *The Holy Bible, English Standard Version*. ESV® Permanent Text Edition® (2016). Copyright © 2001 by Crossway Bibles, a publishing ministry of Good News Publishers.
4 Choderlos de Laclos, Pierre Ambroise Francois. *Les Liasions Dangerous (Texte E Tabli Sur Le Manuscrit Autographe)*. Paris, 1966.
5 Nin, Anaïs. *In Favor of the Sensitive Man and Other Essays* (Original Harvest Book; Hb333) (Kindle Locations 556-559). Houghton Mifflin Harcourt. Kindle Edition.

Chapter 17: Loss of Feminine Love

1 Benton, Catherine. *God of Desire: Tales of Kaĺ Madeva in Sanskrit Story Literature*. Albany, State University of New York Press, 2006, p. 31.
2 *The Poetry of Arnaut Daniel*. Translated by James J. Wilhelm. London, Taylor & Francis, 1983.

3 Kehew, Robert, et al. *Lark in the Morning the Verses of the Troubadours: A Bilingual Edition*. Chicago, University of Chicago Press, 2005.

4 Ibid.

5 Ibid.

6 Neruda, Pablo, and Ilan Stavans. "I Do Not Love You Except Because I Love You." *The Poetry of Pablo Neruda*. New York, Farrar, Straus and Giroux, 2005.

Chapter 18: Cheating: It's Not All About Sex

1 Malachi 2:13–14. *New American Standard Bible*. Copyright ©1960, 1962, 1963, 1968, 1971, 1972, 1973, 1975, 1977, 1995 by The Lockman Foundation, La Habra, Calif. All rights reserved.

2 Coelho, Paulo, and Susan Denaker. *Adultery*. Tullamarine, Australia, Bolinda Publishing Pty Ltd, 2015.

3 Neuman, M. Gary. *The Truth about Cheating: Why Men Stray and What You Can Do to Prevent It*. Turner Publishing Company. Kindle Edition, p 16,

4 Ibid.

5 Ibid.

6 Ibid.

7 Ibid.

8 Ibid.

9 Wallace, Kelly. "Study: Men with Breadwinning Wives More Likely to Cheat." *CNN*, Cable News Network, 1 June 2015, www.cnn.com/2015/06/01/living/infidelity-men-women-breadwinners-feat/index.html.

10 Neuman, *The Truth about Cheating: Why Men Stray and What You Can Do to Prevent It*.

11 Boteach, Rabbi Shmuley. "Why Men Cheat and How They Can Be Stopped." *The Huffington Post*, TheHuffingtonPost.com, 17 December 2009, www.huffingtonpost.com/Rabbi-shmuley-boteach/why-men-cheat-and-how-the_b_394750.html.

12 Neruda, Pablo, and Donald Devenish Walsh. "If You Forget Me." *Love Poems*. New York, New Directions Paperbacks, 2008.

Chapter 19: Unavailability

1 Bryant, William Cullen. "View from the Euganean Hills, North Italy," Percy Bysshe Shelley. *New Library of Poetry and Song Volume 1*. Rarebooksclub.com, 2012.

2 Mann, Thomas, and David Luke. *Death in Venice and Other Stories*. New York, Vintage Classics, 2010,

3 Song of Songs 3:1–3. Holy Bible, New International Version®, NIV® Copyright ©1973, 1978, 1984, 2011 by Biblical Inc.® Used by permission. All rights reserved worldwide.

4 Fitzgerald, F. Scott. *The Great Gatsby*. New York, Penguin Books, 2000. iBooks.

5 Ibid.

Chapter 20: Mystery

1 Neruda, Pablo. "Ode To a Naked Beauty." *Love Poems*. New York, New Directions Book, 2008.

Chapter 21: Forbiddenness

1. Nin, Anaïs. *The Diary of Anaïs Nin*. Vol. 1 (1931–1934). New York, Houghton Mifflin Harcourt. Kindle Edition.
2. Nin, Anaïs. *Incest: From a Journal of Love, the Unexpurgated Diary … 1932–1934*. P. Owen, 1993.
3. Kierkegaard, Søren. *The Sickness unto Death*. Merchant Books, 2013. iBooks.
4. Popova, Maria. "Philosopher Erich Fromm on the Art of Loving and What Is Keeping Us from Mastering It." *Brain Pickings*, 22 March 2016, www.brainpickings.org/2015/10/29/the-art-of-loving-erich-fromm/.

Chapter 22: Vertical Discovery

1. Browning, Elizabeth Barrett. "How Do I Love Thee? (Sonnet 43)." *Poets.org*, Academy of American Poets, 5 July 2016, www.poets.org/poetsorg/poem/how-do-i-love-thee-sonnet-43.
2. Browning, Robert, et al. *The Letters of Robert Browning and Elizabeth Barrett Browning, 1845–1846*. Cambridge, MA, Belknap Press of Harvard University Press, 1969.
3. Ibid.
4. Ibid.
5. Ibid.
6. Ibid.
7. Ginsberg, Allen. "Sunflower Sutra" from *Collected Poems, 1947–1980*. Copyright © 1984 by Allen Ginsberg. Used with the permission of HarperCollins Publishers.
8. Ibid.
9. Ibid.
10. Proverbs 20:27. *Holy Bible, New International Version*®, Copyright © 1973, 1978, 1984, 2011 by Biblica, Inc.® Used by permission. All rights reserved worldwide.
11. Genesis 2:7. *King James Bible*.
12. Liedloff, Jean. *The Continuum Concept*. http://www.continuum-concept.org/reading/JFL-interview.html
13. Ibid.
14. Ibid.

Building Connection

1. Boteach, Shmuley. *Kosher Lust*. Jerusalem, Gefen, 2014. Kindle Edition.

Channeling Your Femininity

1. Greene, Robert. *The Art of Seduction*. Penguin Publishing Group. Kindle Edition.

Parents Are Still Lovers

1. Boteach, Shmuley. *Kosher Adultery: Seduce and Sin with Your Spouse*. Avon, MA, Adams Media Corp., 2002.

INDEX

narcissistic culture, 31, 135, 194
need to be needed, of males, 129, 138
    achievement and career validation for,
        131–132
    infants in-arms experiences and, 133–134
    intimacy seeking and, 130–131
    male complexity in relationships and,
        135–136
    women laughter and sexuality, 136
needs, 10
    denial of sensual, 13–14
    having sex compared to making love, 16
    loneliness and, 11–12
    male sensual, 15
    sex as weapon or punishment and, 16–17
Neruda, Pablo, 136, 194
    on males erotic connection, 155
Neuman, Gary, 163, 164
Newsweek, on sexless marriage, 21
Nin, Anaïs, 4, 19, 146, 171
    on forbiddenness, 195–196
nonphysical cheating, 162

objectification
    depersonalized sex and, 74
    emotional disconnect from, 76–77
    males pressure for selves in, 73
    pornography and, 75, 81
    sexual experts and, 73–77, 81
    sexual revolution impact on, 75
obligation, 49
obscenity, Supreme Court redefinition of, 60
"Ode to A Naked Beauty" (Neruda), 194
O'Donohue, John, 3
"Oh Best of All Nights, Return and Return
        Again" (Laughlin), 117–118
open marriages, 49, 182
oral sex, 70
Orenstein, Peggy, 60
orgasm, 238
    Deida on, 223
    males and, 80–81, 149
    Osho on, 79
    physical, material, emotional and spiritual,
        82
    women and, 81
    women faking, 80

Osco, Bill, 60
Osho, Indian Mystic, 79
overexposure to sex
    from sexual revolution, 77
    women impacted by, 64
overfamiliarity, passion and, 4
oversexualization
    dysfunction from, 63
    girls sexual development and, 64
    hunger for sex and, 86
    males on women attraction and, 64–65

painful intercourse, of women, 110–111
parenting, 7, 241–242
    modeling love for children through, 240
passion
    Liedloff on teaching children, 217
    overfamiliarity and, 4
    for sexual power, 4
passionate connectedness, 140–141, 144, 150
    absence and impact on women, 121–123
    loneliness in marriage and, 116–118
    male absence of, 121–124
    male need for, 143–144
    practice of, 244–249
    women need for, 113–119
patriarchal culture, 27, 102, 103, 159
Percy, Walker, 160
person as unique entity, Fromm on, 73
physical intimacy, 246
    depersonalized sex absence of, 69–70
    instead of emotional connectedness, 16
physical orgasm, 82
physiological response, of women, 105–106
Plante, Rebecca, 134–135
platonic love, 21
polyamory, 49
pornography, 19, 38, 46–47, 53, 192
    addiction to, 140–141, 212
    adultery and, 42
    American Academy of Matrimonial Lawyers
        on, 39–40
    brain changes from, 40, 42
    children impacted by, 44–45
    communication interruption of, 41
    divorce statistics and, 39–40
    drugs and, 65

ABOUT THE AUTHORS

SHMULEY BOTEACH is an American Orthodox rabbi, author, TV host, and public speaker. Known as "America's Rabbi," whom *The Washington Post* and *Newsweek* call "the most famous Rabbi in America," *The Jerusalem Post* lists as one of the fifty most influential Jews in the world, and the *New York Observer* calls "the best-known Orthodox Jew in the world," Shmuley is one of the world's leading values and spirituality exponents and relationship experts. Rabbi Shmuley regularly appears on global TV programs, including guest appearances on *The Oprah Winfrey Show*, *The Dr. Oz Show*, and *The View*; on the radio; and in print media including *The New York Times*, *The Wall Street Journal*, *The Huffington Post*, *The Daily Beast*, and *The Jerusalem Post*.

PAMELA ANDERSON is an internationally recognized model, actress, and philanthropist. She starred in *Baywatch* and appeared on more *Playboy* covers than anyone else in history (fourteen). A long-time supporter of animal rights, Anderson continues to act and advance the work of her foundation. Pamela has nearly 2.5 million followers on Facebook, Instagram, and Twitter. A devoted mother of two, Pamela has distinguished herself as a Hollywood icon who has always emphasized the need for balance of womanhood and motherhood and of individual achievement and communal responsibility.